The Surgical Solution

The Surgical Solution

A History of Involuntary
Sterilization in the United States

Philip R. Reilly, M.D., J.D.

The Johns Hopkins University Press
Baltimore and London

The Johns Hopkins University Press,
701 West 40th Street, Baltimore, Maryland 21211
The Johns Hopkins Press Ltd., London

∞ The paper used in this book meets the minimum requirements of American
National Standard for Information Sciences—Permanence of Paper for Printed
Library Materials, ANSI Z39.48-1984.

Library of Congress Cataloging-in-Publication Data

Reilly, Philip, 1947–
    The surgical solution : a history of involuntary sterilization in the United States / Philip
R. Reilly.
        p.   cm.
    Includes bibliographical references.
    Includes index.
    ISBN 0-8018-4096-1 (alk. paper)
    1. Eugenics—United States—History.   2. Mentally handicapped—Surgery—United
States—History.   I. Title.
    [DNLM: 1. Eugenics—history—United States.   2. Mental Retardation—history—
United States.   3. Public Policy—history—United States.   4. Sterilization, Sexual—
history—United States.
HV 4989 R362s]
HQ7555.5.U5R45   1991   87/97
363.9'7—dc20   1800
DNLM/DLC
for Library of Congress   90-5090

To Sarah Anne Reilly and Thomas Marshall Reilly

Contents

Foreword

In recent decades, historians of medicine have moved beyond the preoccupation with the careers of prominent physicians and the traditional emphasis on the inexorable progress of medical thought and practice. They have begun to ask novel questions and explore hitherto neglected problems: the relationship between medicine and society; the interplay of popular and professional concepts of health and disease; the role of environmental and socioeconomic variables in changing morbidity and mortality patterns; the rise of new institutional forms and systems of treatment and care; and the ways in which medical interventions and technologies were actually employed. In so doing, they have appreciably weakened the older commitment to historicism—the belief that human history is moving on an upward gradient toward an ideal end or purpose. Less concerned with celebrating the progress of medicine, contemporary scholars seek to understand the sources of change and the ways in which the health care system actually worked and the uses to which it was put.

The history of involuntary sterilization provides a dramatic illustration of the inseparable relationship between medicine, on the one hand, and broader social processes, on the other. In the late nineteenth century, a series of currents converged to give rise to the belief that the very character of American society was being threatened by the growing numbers of degenerate persons whose biological traits predisposed them to lives of crime, idleness, poverty, dependency, alcoholism, insanity, idiocy, and disease generally. A faith that culture was shaped by biology rather than environment colored the responses of many Americans who believed that the increase in degeneracy from both indigenous and foreign sources menaced the stability, tranquillity, and well-being of their nation.

By the turn of the century, the pervasive tide of fear had already begun to shape public policies. The segregation of allegedly degenerate persons in institutions was common practice. A nascent restrictionist movement based on the belief that continued immigration of individuals from Eastern and Southern Europe with inferior genes constituted a distinct menace was also taking shape. In such an environment it was hardly surprising that some individuals and groups would enthusiastically support the involuntary sterilization of individuals whose allegedly immoral and undesirable behavior reflected an inferior biological heritage.

The Surgical Solution, by Philip R. Reilly—whose training in medicine and history has sensitized him to the complexities of social processes—represents the first scholarly effort to focus on the origins and history of involuntary sterilization. As he clearly demonstrates, the development of vasectomy (and, subsequently, salpingectomy) was from the very beginning wedded to a faith that medical science had within its grasp a simple but humane procedure that would not deform the individual and would benefit society. Indeed, involuntary sterilization represented an effort to uplift society by preventing the propagation of persons whose socially undesirable behavior supposedly resulted from a deficient biological inheritance. That sterilization had considerable appeal was demonstrated by the fact that about two-thirds of all states enacted legislation legitimating the procedure in one form or another.

The subsequent history of involuntary sterilization, as Dr. Reilly so well points out, was more complex than is generally realized. By World War I, many of the early statutes had ceased to be effective. During the 1920s and 1930s—decades during which xenophobia toward racial and ethnic groups enjoyed a resurgence—involuntary sterilization gained a new life. Led by Harry H. Laughlin, a small but effective group of supporters that included prominent physicians promoted the passage of laws designed to protect the purity of America's racial heritage. Nor was sterilization a verbal symbol; in the Great Depression years, about twenty-five hundred individuals underwent this radical procedure annually. Germany was one of the few other nations to follow the American example in adopting legislation providing for mandatory sterilization of groups designated as defective.

But the most striking part of Dr. Reilly's history is his description of the post–World War II decades. During the war, the number of involuntary sterilizations (as compared with those performed in the 1930s) declined rapidly, largely because so many able-bodied surgeons had been inducted into the military. The return of peace saw a partial resurgence of sterilization despite clear knowledge and evidence of Nazi practices and experiments. Interestingly enough, the subsequent decline of sterilization for eugenic purposes was accompanied by efforts to make elective sterilization an option for controlling family size. Yet, involuntary sterilization—challenges to its constitutionality notwithstanding—did not disappear altogether. Indeed, available data suggest that involuntary sterilization continues to attract the allegiance of some persons who perceive it as an effective way of dealing with pressing social problems.

What can we learn from the origins, rise, and decline of eugenic sterilization? The "lessons" of history, to be sure, are generally obscure and frequently contradictory. Moreover, those who use history to justify their own prescriptions invariably select examples that prove their case and ignore all data to the contrary. After 1945, for example, cold war warriors generally employed the analogy of Munich to support their argument for a diplomacy that rested on military strength. The weaknesses of Western democracies in the 1930s, they insisted, encouraged Hitler and his Nazi supporters in their aggressive ways and thus made the outbreak of World War II a certainty. Yet, the very same individuals who argued that military preparedness was a prerequisite for peace ignored the example of World War I. In 1914, all of the major European powers were militarily prepared, and yet war—not peace—followed.

To suggest that the lessons of history are unclear, however, is not to argue that the study of the past is futile. On the contrary, the study of the past illuminates the limitations that serve to define the very character of human beings. The practice of involuntary sterilization, after all, did not arise solely from evil or selfish motives. On the contrary, its advocates were persuaded that they were acting on behalf of a noble cause that would benefit humanity. They believed that medical and scientific knowledge, combined with a new technology, had reached a point in time in which the eradication of inherited defects was possible. That their belief in their own omniscience was flawed is, of course, a truism. Yet the dream of human mastery remains an alluring possibility, whether expressed in religious, scientific, or medical terminology. Because individuals act on the basis of their beliefs, this Faustian dream is unlikely to be without consequences. In this sense, Dr. Reilly's history of involuntary sterilization in the United States should force us to question all claims of omniscience—religious, scientific, medical—lest we follow in the steps of our predecessors and inflict endless suffering on others.

Gerald N. Grob

Preface

The history of involuntary sterilization is but one aspect of the history of eugenics in the United States. I do not pretend to take on the larger subject, once one of the nation's major intellectual preoccupations, so ably addressed by Mark Haller, Kenneth Ludmerer, Daniel Kevles, Garland Allen, Bentley Glass, and other historians.

During the first six decades of the twentieth century, more than sixty thousand mentally retarded or mentally ill individuals, most of them residents of large state institutions, were sterilized for eugenic reasons. Even the most accommodating view of sterilization programs must recognize that at best only a tiny fraction of such persons consented to the surgery. Indeed, hundreds and possibly thousands of people, most of them women, were never told that they had been sterilized. It is extraordinary how many "appendectomies" were performed at some state homes for the retarded in the 1920s and 1930s.

Today, a report that a single retarded person had been involuntarily sterilized would evoke much attention from both the newspapers and the courts. Clearly, much has changed.

I set out to reconstruct and document the rise and decline of eugenic sterilization programs in the United States. How did they come about? What were the concerns of the legislators in the many states that adopted sterilization laws? Who were the lobbyists? Who drafted the bills? Once the laws had been enacted, who set up the programs? What were the criteria for sterilization? Did the criteria change over time? Were there significant differences in the operation of such programs? Did they vary by institution, by state, by region? What stimulated their expansion?

If assessed simply by the number of persons sterilized each year, the programs reached their zenith in the late 1930s. They then entered a long, slow decline, punctuated by increasing activity in at least one geographical region. What caused the decline? Why did sterilization programs persist (contrary to many assertions) well after World War II? Are retarded persons still sterilized today?

I have been able to answer some of the questions. Along the way I have learned that the dignity of mentally retarded and mentally ill persons was systematically ignored in the United States for many decades. This book, which documents a sad history of the nation's abuse of retarded persons and others, also indicates how much the notion of personal autonomy has matured in our society.

Acknowledgments

One of the requirements for graduation from Yale Medical School is to write a thesis. While I was a student at Yale I had the good fortune to be a student of Thomas Forbes, a professor of anatomy with a deep interest in the history of medicine. His informal seminars on Vesalius, Paré, and others fascinated me. When it was time to take on the thesis project, I chose to study the role played by physicians in the American eugenics movement, and Dr. Forbes agreed to act as my adviser. That thesis was the kernel of this work.

Unquestionably, the most enjoyable part of this effort was the many days spent (both before and after my graduation) working in archives. My investigations led me to the American Philosophical Society in Philadelphia, the Rockefeller Archive in Tarrytown, New York, the Social Welfare History Archive at the University of Minnesota in Minneapolis, the Minnesota Historical Society in St. Paul, the Connecticut State Library in Hartford, Rice University in Houston, and the Pickler Memorial Library at Northeast Missouri State University in Kirksville. There were also fruitful visits to the New York Academy of Medicine, the New York Public Library, and the Library of Congress. Of course, I also made extensive use of materials held by the Yale libraries. The one common thread in these travels was the courtesy and helpfulness of archivists and librarians too numerous to mention.

My study is primarily concerned with the history of involuntary sterilization of institutionalized retarded persons. My research led me to visit several large institutions, including the Faribault State School in Faribault, Minnesota, Lynchburg Colony in Lynchburg, Virginia, the State Training School in Mansfield, Connecticut, and the Fernald State School in Waltham, Massachusetts. Interviews with individuals working at these institutions greatly enriched my knowledge of what life was like for retarded persons residing at such places fifty years ago.

Garland Allen and Bentley Glass, two scholars who have far greater knowledge of the history of eugenics than do I, offered helpful advice.

xv

Glass suggested many changes for an article based on a portion of this work that appeared several years ago in the *Quarterly Review of Biology*. Margery Shaw, who introduced me to the field of human genetics, read early drafts of the book and provided much encouragement. Joanne Cusack and Eileen McClellan were invaluable in helping me prepare the manuscript.

My wife, Nancy, always a good listener, helped me shape this story. She joined me in several rather odd vacations that found us visiting libraries or institutions for the mentally retarded rather than theaters or resorts.

The Surgical Solution

1 · The Heritability of Degeneracy

> It is a reproach to our intelligence that we as a people, proud in other respects of our control of nature, should have to support about half a million insane, feeble-minded, epileptic, blind and deaf, 80,000 prisoners and 100,000 paupers at a cost of over 100 million dollars per year.
>
> —C. B. Davenport, *Heredity in Relation to Eugenics*, 1911

> Stories about a few men who had or were presumed to have an extra Y chromosome and who had committed serious crimes were given prominent attention in the press, suggesting the intriguing idea that the single Y chromosome normally found in males contributes to aggressive tendencies in that sex and that an extra Y carries these tendencies beyond their usual bounds.
>
> —H. A. Witkin et al., "XYY and XXY Men: Criminality and Aggression," *Science*, 1976

During the last quarter of the nineteenth century, it was widely believed that many of the social problems that burdened American towns and cities were caused by the misbehavior of degenerate persons, individuals whose biological origins predisposed or even predestined them to lives of crime, poverty, and prostitution. America was still essentially rural in character, and Americans tolerated the village idiots and town drunks, feared the epileptics and insane, supported poorhouses for the destitute and retarded, and preached against vice and alcohol abuse. By the beginning of the twentieth century, nearly every state operated large, centralized, tax-supported institutions for the retarded, the insane, and the epileptic. As the nation became more urban and as bemused tolerance for "degenerates" faded, a policy of segregation flourished. But this was not all. As the perception that such persons constituted a social menace spread, efforts to control and limit their reproduction emerged. This campaign received its ultimate expression in involuntary sterilization, the subject of this book.

Between 1907 and 1960 more than sixty thousand retarded and mentally ill persons were sterilized without their consent, all victims of programs designed to cut off the flow of allegedly defective genes into the nation's gene pool.

It was during a period of growing concern for the menace of the feeble-minded that three European scientists, Carl Correns, Hugo DeVries, and Erich von Tschermark, discovered and confirmed Gregor Mendel's breeding experiments with garden peas. Mendel's work demonstrated the particulate nature of the gene and delineated the basic laws of inheritance, creating the foundation for the science of genetics.[1] The new genetics had great appeal, especially to a few who thought it might provide a solution to the problem of degeneracy, as crime and immorality were commonly labeled.

In addition to advances in genetics, several other important developments also predisposed people to think that complex human behaviors were determined by inheritance. Developments in biology, anthropology, and criminology were especially influential in the rise of involuntary sterilization programs. Unquestionably, the publication of Charles Darwin's great book, *Origin of Species*, in 1859 split the bulwark of resistance to a biological view of humanity. After a century of challenge, biblical time gave way to a vastly longer scientific calendar. Although *Origin of Species* did not focus on humans, Darwin's theory of evolution was universal, and the conclusion that the human species had evolved under natural selection was inescapable. The mechanism of inheritance was not a key feature of Darwin's evolutionary theory; indeed, his speculation that "gemmules" coalesced in the reproductive glands to shape the next generation was merely one of many creative but erroneous notions about heredity that percolated through the nineteenth century. Nevertheless, Darwin altered the way in which people thought about themselves.

The Origin of the Eugenics Movement

The founding father of human genetics was Francis Galton. Around the time that Darwin (his cousin) published *Origin of Species*, Galton was becoming interested in human inheritance. While Darwin's work surely accelerated that interest, there were other factors. Galton's infertile marriage, as well as the infertility of several other marriages within his and his wife's family, was surely one. Relevant intellectual influences included Herbert Spencer, whose notions about the survival of the fittest preceded Darwin's work, and Thomas Malthus, whose mathematical modeling of populations was well known in midcentury England.

In 1864 Galton initiated a study of the frequency with which relatives of eminent men themselves achieved eminence. He published his findings under the title "Hereditary Talent" in the popular *Macmillan's Magazine* in June and August 1865. Galton, who was greatly impressed by the extraordinary number of relatives of eminent men who had also achieved eminence, steadily expanded his inquiry. In 1869 he published a book titled *Hereditary Genius: An Inquiry into Its Laws and Consequences,* in which he stated the bias that would become the cornerstone of the eugenics movement three decades later. Galton wrote:

> I have no patience with the hypothesis occasionally expressed, and often implied, especially in tales written to teach children to be good, that babies are born pretty much alike, and that the sole agencies in creating differences between boy and boy, and man and man are steady application and moral effort. It is in the most unqualified manner that I object to pretensions of natural equality. The experiences of the nursery, the school, the university, and of professional careers, are a chain of proofs to the contrary.[2]

Galton was not without his critics. Alphonse de Candolle, a Swiss scientist, published *Histoire des sciences et des savants depuis deux siècles* (1871), a work that accused Galton of overstating the importance of heredity. This stimulated Galton to launch more studies. With advice from Herbert Spencer, he prepared a long questionnaire covering topics such as family characteristics, body build, temperament, education, and religious beliefs that he asked 180 members of the Royal Society, Great Britain's most prestigious scientific body, to answer. Using data collected from 100 respondents, he prepared his next book, *English Men of Science: Their Nature and Nurture* (1874), a work that seemed to prove his thesis that talent was largely determined by heredity. The data showed that of the 660 men who were closely related to the 100 respondents, 13 were *eminent,* a category that, by Galton's criteria, was deserved by no more than 50 of all the men who died in that nation each year.[3]

During the century's last two decades, Galton, a classic Victorian intellectual who published broadly and tirelessly, devoted much of his attention to anthropometry. He was a man obsessed with measuring. He measured phenomena as diverse as cutaneous flush during excitement and the efficacy of prayer to help heal the sick.[4] The mass of data that Galton compiled helped to probe the nature-nurture problem ever more deeply. By 1883, when he published *Inquiries into Human Faculty and Its Development,* Galton was convinced that humankind could modify and improve its own species, a policy for which he coined a new word, "eugenics." Even though he acknowledged that the subject was "entangled with collateral considerations," Galton offered the first ideas on how to implement eugenic policies.[5]

From 1883 until his death in 1911, Galton generated a steady flow of articles on eugenics. In 1904 he donated money to the University of London to start a Eugenics Record Office. In so doing he sought recognition of an official definition of "natural eugenics," which after some modifications by a university committee, emerged as "the study of the agencies under social control that may improve or impair the racial qualities of future generations either physically or mentally."[6]

Although he is recognized as the founder of the eugenics movement, it is difficult to estimate Galton's impact on American thought. He never visited the United States. Neither of his books on eugenics sold well in England or the United States. He did contribute several articles on eugenics to American periodicals, but by the time they appeared there were already many Americans who espoused eugenic principles. But, given his place in Victorian society, there can be little doubt that Galton's work conferred a large measure of intellectual respectability on the "science" of eugenics.

The late nineteenth century was a period of rapid advance in biology, and the work of several other important scientists helped, however unintentionally, to create a favorable climate for eugenics. For example, in the 1880s the German biologist August Weismann reached his revolutionary conclusions about the continuity of the germ plasm. This thesis rang the death knell for the Lamarckian notion that acquired abilities could be passed on.[7] Several decades later eugenicists would regularly argue that aberrant social behavior ran in families because of tainted genes. Another important contribution came from Ernst Haeckel, a professor of anatomy at the University of Jena in Switzerland, who applied Darwin's ideas to explain the evolution of humans. Convinced that man had descended from an earlier hominid, Haeckel pushed God's hand farther back in time.[8]

Herbert Spencer was also extremely influential. As Richard Hofstadter wrote, "In the three decades after the Civil War it was impossible to be active in any field of intellectual work without mastering Spencer."[9] From the *Synthetic Philosophy* (1864) to the less weighty and widely read *Study of Sociology,* which appeared in serial form in the *Popular Science Monthly* during the early 1870s, Spencer refined his unique view of the implication of evolutionary theory for human society. As early as 1850 his *Social Statistics* bluntly stated ideas that would appeal to the eugenics movement fifty years later. As Spencer put it, "Nature" was a great court in which people were tried: "If they are sufficiently complete to live, they do live, and it is well they should live. If they are not sufficiently complete to live, they die and it is best they should die."[10] In a society that embraced this idea, programs to curb reproduction by the feeble-minded would hardly seem to constitute a radical violation of rights.

Evolutionary Theory and Racial Differences

Despite a strong theological resistance to the Darwinian thesis, many Americans were drawn into its grasp. One attraction was the implication that evolutionary theory held for race relations. For whatever harm it did to biblical cosmology, the theory of natural selection had the benefit of providing a method with which to rationalize the widely held belief that the Negro was inferior to the Caucasian. From its birth the United States, a country of red and white and black (and, by the late nineteenth century, yellow), had struggled painfully with the problems of racial inequality. How could slavery be maintained in a nation that had been conceived on the principle that "all men are created equal"? Though the Civil War ended slavery, it did not change racial attitudes. It is hardly surprising that nine teenth-century Americans were deeply interested in the origin of races.

Of course, speculation about human differences has been a perennial topic for reflection. What is unique about the nineteenth century is that Scripture was rejected as the authoritative word on human typology, giving way to physical measurements of human variability. When the century began, the monogenist view that all humankind belonged to a single species dominated. For Buffon and Kant and most of their colleagues, the ability of persons of different races to breed successfully provided an incontrovertible proof. Of course, even the most freethinking naturalist believed that God had made humankind.

It was still necessary, however, to explain the physical and cultural differences between peoples in northwestern Europe, coastal Africa, and Central America. Many leading thinkers, particularly the Comte de Buffon, the author of *Histoire naturelle* (1749), and Johann Blumenbach (1752-1840), a German anatomist, believed that human races had been produced by *degeneration* from an original type. Color provided a rough index of the degree of degeneration. The concept of racial degeneration satisfied the conviction shared by Europeans and North Americans of their innate superiority without violating the Old Testament. If God had made a single, perfect human, only degeneration could explain the "obvious" physical inferiority and cultural weakness of the African.[11] A century later, American eugenicists would argue that insanity and feeble-mindedness were expressions of mental degeneracy and that criminals were moral degenerates. This made it easier to label them as inferior and to invoke sterilization programs to deal with them.

In the United States, perhaps the earliest expositor of the monogenist view was the Reverend Samuel Stanhope Smith, a professor of moral philosophy at Princeton. His treatise titled *Essay on the Causes of the Variety of Complexion and Figure in the Human Species* (1787), which eschewed the notion of degeneration in favor of variation, ascribed obvious racial differences to the impact of environment over the centuries. In trying to explain how environmental influences became hereditary, he clung to a crude version of Lamarckism. Noting that the sun caused light-skinned people to freckle, Dr. Smith speculated that Negroes might inherit a "universal freckle." Dr. Benjamin Rush, a leading physician in colonial America, agreed that racial differences were environmentally induced. He thought that dark skin predisposed to leprosy. Rush opposed miscegenation, fearing that it would transfer a susceptibility to leprosy to American whites.[12]

The first major American challenge to the thesis that races had arisen from a common type came in 1839 when Dr. Samuel George Morton, a Philadelphia physician, published *Crania Americana*. Morton, who had been taught that the world's age could be derived from Scripture, was troubled by evidence provided by Egyptologists that the Negro and Caucasian were already distinct during the reign of the Pharaohs. Biologists had demonstrated that species changed slowly, so how could there have been sufficient time for the necessary divergence (or degeneration) from a common type between Eden and Egypt? Morton concluded that the Bible was not literally true and that after the Flood different races must have emerged, blessed by God with features adapted to their home climates.[13]

Morton sought to explore racial differences by conducting a systematic physical examination of 256 skulls from five major peoples (Caucasian, Mongolian, Malay, American, and Ethiopian). Proceeding with what appeared to be sound scientific caution, he used lead shot to measure the volume of each cranium. He found that there were significant differences in cranial capacity among the different peoples. Although he at first hesitated to draw the inference that his findings could be used to distinguish the races, by 1840 Morton was certain that the average capacity of the Caucasian skull was seven cubic inches greater than that of the Negro skull. As he had firmly rejected an environmentalist explanation for this variance, and as Darwin had yet to publish his revolutionary thesis, Morton had no choice but to conclude that the Creator had varied cranial size among the races. The findings were reassuring: if Caucasians had bigger brains, were not they superior? Had not God so ordained? Only recently has the eminent Harvard paleontologist Stephen Jay Gould shown that Morton's measurements were significantly biased.[14]

Among other early scientific studies of racial inequality, one based on the 1840 census is noteworthy. This census (the sixth) was the first to enumerate "insane persons" and "idiots." Dr. Edward Jarvis, a Harvard-trained physician who had grown interested in vital statistics, analyzed those data for the Census Bureau and found that there was a much higher prevalence of insanity among Negroes in the North than in the South. This led him to publish a paper speculating that slavery, not freedom, was more conducive to the black man's tranquillity.[15] On reexamination, however, Jarvis discovered that reports of insanity among Negroes in some northern cities were so high as to be preposterous. Although he quickly published a paper refuting his own findings, the damage was done. For the rest of his life, Jarvis, who became an authority on the United States census, sought unsuccessfully to have Congress reject the official report from 1840.[16]

Among the problems that most troubled those who were convinced of the distinctiveness and inferiority of blacks, none was more troubling than miscegenation. One major proponent of the thesis that the mulatto was vastly inferior to white *and* black was Dr. Josiah Nott. Nott, a South Carolinian who had earned his medical degree at the University of Pennsylvania in 1827, published his first dire warnings in 1843. The paper, which predicted the ultimate extermination of both races in favor of the degenerate mulatto, argued that Caucasian and Negro were separate species. Dr. Nott believed that God engaged in several acts of creation, one for each race. His observations as a physician drew him to the conviction that the mulatto would always be inferior to either racial progenitor.[17] The protection of racial integrity became Nott's mission in life. For twenty years he argued that different races had arisen independently, a view that clearly supported assertions of inequality. One of his more influential acts was to translate Arthur Gobineau's *Essai sur l'inequalité des races humaines* (1853), a work that presaged later American concerns about the impact of immigrants of weak racial stock on the nation's biological vigor. Nott dedicated the book to "the Statesmen of America."[18]

The argument that blacks were inferior to whites and that miscegenation was dangerous was widespread during the latter half of the nineteenth century. By the end of the century, many whites believed that evolution had led the Caucasian to intelligence, culture, and civilization, while the Negro had progressed only very slowly or, possibly, even degenerated from more successful ancestors. Such thinking could easily tolerate assertions of inferiority and degeneracy in other groups, including the feeble-minded, an attitude that helped lead to the decision to sterilize so many of them.

The Heritability of Deviance

The last twenty years of the nineteenth century also saw a steady growth in the number of proponents of a biological basis for feeble-mindedness, epilepsy, insanity, and crime. There were, however, relatively few scientific studies to support such theories. One important exception was in criminal anthropology. For nearly fifty years, beginning with his studies of Italian soldiers in 1864, Cesare Lombroso, the founder of the positivist school of criminology, investigated the physical anthropology of hundreds of criminals. Although he proposed an extraordinary number of sensible ideas (such as liberal divorce laws to reduce crimes of adultery), Lombroso's most famous work was based on now-discredited anthropomorphic studies that were once widely accepted in the United States.

By his own account, Lombroso's notion of the "born" criminal was a flash of insight. During an autopsy of a famous brigand named Vilella, Lombroso noticed an unusual depression not found in normal human skulls (a median occipital fossa) but commonly seen in rodent skulls. This was not merely an idea but a revelation. At the sight of that skull, he seemed to see all of a sudden, "lighted up as a vast plain under a flaming sky, the problem of the nature of the criminal—an atavistic being who reproduces in his person the ferocious instincts of primitive humanity and the inferior animals."[19]

Soon thereafter, while interviewing a mass murderer named Misdea, who had epilepsy, "which appeared to be hereditary in all the members of his family," Lombroso had a second revelation:

> It flashed across my mind that many criminal characteristics not attributable to atavism, such as facial asymmetry, cerebral sclerosis, impulsiveness, instantaneousness, the periodicity of criminal acts, the desire for evil for evil's sake, were morbid characteristics common to epilepsy, mingled with others due to atavism.[20]

Lombroso's ideas that atavism and morbid characteristics were major causes of crime were powerful forces in American criminological and medical thought in the 1890s. In *Prisoners and Paupers* (1893), the criminologist Henry M. Boies, a member of the Pennsylvania Board of Public Charities and the State Committee on Lunacy, asserted:

> Everyone who has visited prisons and observed large numbers of prisoners together has undoubtedly been impressed from the appearance of prisoners alone, that a large portion of them were born to be criminals. There would seem to be certain recognizable features which differentiate these from the

rest of mankind, and set them apart as a criminal class, of which it might be assumed that, although any given individual might be reclaimed and saved, as a class the whole were destined to live and die criminals.[21]

Later in the same work, Boies articulated the tenets of biological determination that would soon generate a call for action: "The laws of biology, that like begets like, that imperfect seed in parentage cannot produce perfect offspring, that breeding in intensifies and magnifies parental peculiarities, that certain inherited defects or deficiencies induce criminality, and result in pauperism, are well-known, and generally accepted to be as invariable and immutable as the law of gravitation."[22]

Although such scholarly works were influential, they reached a relatively small audience. In seeking to understand why the eugenics movement flourished in America and, particularly, the reasons why so many states implemented programs to sterilize persons perceived to be defective, one must accord special weight to a single study of a New York family conducted by a transplanted Englishman named Richard Dugdale.

During the late 1860s and 1870s, Dugdale, whose inheritance permitted him to pursue a zealous interest in social reform, was extremely active in New York City. He was (often simultaneously) the secretary of the Section on Sociology of the New York Association for the Advancement of Science and the Arts, of the New York Social Science Society, and of the New York Sociological Club; treasurer of the New York Liberal Club; and vice-president of the Society for the Prevention of Street Accidents. In 1868 he became a member of the Executive Committee of the New York Prison Association. While working with that group he met Dr. Elisha Harris, a physician who was its corresponding secretary. In 1874 Harris persuaded him to assist in inspecting county jails, and Dugdale agreed to cover the northern part of the state. Their objective was to study prisoners in order to acquire a more sophisticated understanding of what had led them to commit crimes and how the circle of recidivism could be broken.[23] Harris and Dugdale developed a detailed survey that included questions on heredity, family history, education, medical history, and "moral and intellectual capacity." Although he had taken courses in business and sociology at Cooper Union, Dugdale had no university training. However, he had read Malthus, and he was an early advocate of birth control. It is likely that in the summer of 1874 he carried two intellectual convictions with his questionnaire into the county jails: a Malthusian concern for overpopulation and a Lombrosian notion that some criminals owed their fate to heredity.

While interviewing prisoners in one jail, Dugdale realized that six of them were related. He became fascinated by their family, and he redirected his efforts to an exhaustive study of its interaction with the state's criminal justice and rudimentary social welfare system. Beginning with the six prisoners, Dugdale eventually traced the lives of 709 persons who were related by blood (540) or marriage or cohabitation (169) to five sisters who had married the sons of one Max, a descendant of Dutch settlers who had been born around 1730. Nicknaming them the "Jukes," he traced the family "with more or less exactness through five generations." He concluded that the Jukes had an extraordinary propensity for the almshouses, prisons, and brothels of New York. Although Dugdale thought that a complicated interplay of environment and heredity accounted for the family's failure to live normal, productive lives, he was intrigued by the genetic component. For example, he speculated that "harlotry may become a hereditary characteristic and be perpetuated without any specially favoring environment to call it into activity."[24]

It is not easy to reconstruct Dugdale's theory of heredity, but he was essentially a Lamarckian. His belief that characteristics could be acquired and perpetuated was embellished by his notion that inbreeding and outbreeding could reinforce or diminish a trait and that reversions to prior types in the line could occur. Although Dugdale ascribed great importance to heredity, he also acknowledged that in some areas environment was key. He believed that "where the conduct depends on the knowledge of moral obligation (excluding insanity and idiocy), the environment has more influence than the heredity because the development of the moral attributes is mainly a postnatal and not an antenatal formation of cerebral cells."[25]

In disseminating his views, Dugdale failed to anticipate that the public would ignore his relatively complex analysis and instead would seize the fact that he had described five *generations* of paupers and criminals. Of course, the title of his first publicly delivered address, "Hereditary Pauperism as Illustrated in the Juke Family," delivered to the American Social Science Association in the fall of 1877, did little to dispel the views of those who preferred a hereditarian explanation.[26] In 1877, George W. Putnam, a publisher who had worked on several committees with Dugdale, published *The Jukes*. It was an immediate success, going through three printings in several months.

The Jukes provided powerful evidence to those persons who believed that aberrant or deviant behavior (crime, intemperance, prostitution) was biologically determined. The social welfare literature of the eighties abounds with references to the Jukes family. It spawned a new social science genre that reached its height four decades later when numerous other eugenicists, particularly Charles B. Davenport and his colleagues at Cold Spring Harbor, conducted studies modeled after Dugdale's work. *The Tribe of Ishmael* (1888), *The Hill Folk* (1912), *The Nam Family* (1912), *The Kallikaks* (1912), and *Dwellers in the Vale of Siddem* (1919) were instrumental in rationalizing the arguments favoring lifetime segregation of defective persons, the Victorian solution to the propagation problem. These studies argued that defectives were unusually fecund and that they cost society a fortune for institutional care. This greatly reinforced the argument for lifetime institutionalization and set the stage for eugenic sterilization programs.

2 · The Cost of Degeneracy

> Over a million and a quarter dollars of loss in 75 years, caused by a single family 1,200 strong, without reckoning the cash paid for whiskey, or taking into account the entailment of pauperism and crime of the survivors in succeeding generations, and the incurable disease, idiocy, and insanity growing out of this debauchery, and reaching further than we can calculate.
>
> —Richard L. Dugdale, *The Jukes,* 1877

> A conservative research institution here (the Heritage Foundation) has just published the factually preposterous and morally repulsive thought that a key reason why academic achievement standards have fallen is that the federal government has dismantled an academically demanding curriculum by catering to special interest groups such as the handicapped, and has favored the disadvantaged pupils at the expense of those who have the highest potential to contribute positively to society.
>
> —George F. Will, "A Magna Carta for the Handicapped," *Boston Globe,* June 23, 1983

Among the first American institutions dedicated to the care of the feeble-minded were those started in Massachusetts in 1848. During the 1850s, proponents of institutional care and training for persons who might otherwise live as village idiots secured legislative support in New York (1851), Pennsylvania (1853), Connecticut (1855), Ohio (1857), and Kentucky (1860). The Civil War caused a hiatus, but a number of new institutions also opened in the 1870s. At first, most arguments in favor of state-supported institutions were largely altruistic. But during the 1870s the superintendents of these institutions enhanced their appeals for legislative support by arguing that money spent on the so-called schools was a wise investment that would reduce the social burden of crime, prostitution, and illegitimacy that would be incurred by failing to isolate the feeble-minded.[1]

The pace of building state-supported institutions for feeble-minded youth was still brisk in the 1880s. Between 1876 and 1885 Iowa, Minnesota, Indiana, Kansas, California, and Nebraska joined the northeastern states and Illinois in opening such schools. The economically devastated southern states did not begin to support such institutions for another decade. By 1888 there were fifteen institutions in fourteen states caring for 4,216 pupils. As early as 1877 the community of persons devoted to the care of the mentally retarded was large enough to create and sustain a national organization, the Association of Medical Officers of American Institutions for Idiotic and Feeble-minded Persons (AMO), the forerunner of today's American Association on Mental Retardation (AAMR).

The AMO annual reports chronicle the shifts in the support offered to these schools by the states. For example, in 1878 Dr. Hervey B. Wilbur, director of the State Asylum for Idiots in Syracuse, proudly reported to his colleagues that the "legislature ha[d] never failed to grant reasonable requests for funds."[2] Similarly, the medical director of Ohio's Institution for Feeble-minded Youth asserted that "our institution holds a warm place in the hearts of our people." The state had provided him with $180,000 "to spend in any way we see fit" on the care and training of 324 pupils in the Ohio institution.[3]

Legislative support for the institutions remained strong in the eighties, but concern for the costs of such institutional care was growing. As early as 1880 Dr. Isaac Kerlin, medical director at Elwyn, Pennsylvania, and the nation's leading physician in the field of mental retardation, warned that "the state will not burden taxpayers with the support of more than a fraction" of the nation's feeble-minded. Given the data reported by the 1880 census, Kerlin's concern was justified. There was an "idiotic population" of 76,895, of whom only 2,429 were in public institutions. It was no surprise that every state institution had a long waiting list. According to Kerlin, the general population had increased by 30 percent in ten years, but the "apparent" increase in idiocy was 200 percent. Further, he was convinced that the census had seriously underestimated the feeble-minded. Of the 295 retarded children for whom application for admission to Elwyn had been made in 1880, Kerlin noted that fewer than half had been listed in the census.[4]

Curbing Reproduction by the Feeble-Minded

It was during 1880 that the AMO first formally considered a program to reduce the propagation of the unfit. A year earlier Amy Shaw Lowell, a prominent New Yorker, had successfully lobbied to start a women's asylum in Newark, New York. The legislature had shown "no hesitation" in providing $15,000 to start this project. Because the funds were to be spent to house and protect ninety-seven "weak minded females," many of whom had borne illegitimate children and who were "life-long burdens upon the tax-payers," it seemed like a wise expenditure. The Newark asylum, intended to protect women who were "so simple as to be easily led away by designing men," represented a shift in the approach to the feeble-minded that troubled some members of the AMO. Until 1879 the primary emphasis in New York had been on intensive training of the feeble-minded in order to return them to a self-supporting status in society. Unlike the larger state schools, Newark did not emphasize programs to train the women. In effect, it incarcerated women primarily to protect them from becoming pregnant.[5]

During the 1880s, other experts concluded that many weak-minded persons were untrainable, and the AMO reports note a steady addition of "custodial" departments to these schools. But planning for lifetime care meant an increase in budgetary needs. The institutions moved quickly to become self-supporting. There was a friendly competition between them as the superintendents bragged of dairy farms, vegetable gardens, shoe factories, and the like.

By the late 1880s the growth in the number of institutions had slowed, waiting lists were longer, and new buildings were filling rapidly. The importance of segregating feeble-minded persons, especially women during their reproductive years, was now openly and frequently discussed. In commenting upon the Newark Asylum for Women, which now housed three hundred "girls" and had obtained funding to house an additional one hundred, one expert urged that "we owe it not only to the adult imbecile herself, but to humanity and the world at large to guard in every possible way against the abuse and increase of this class." At least one New York official was convinced that a policy of lifetime incarceration would work. In his view there was no doubt that "the propagation of idiocy, which was formerly carried on through the medium of this class of weak-minded girls among the homes and poor-houses of our State, will henceforth be materially lessened." Similar comments suggest that there was unwarranted optimism that by segregating a few thousand simple-minded women, society could stem a significant fraction of the births of defective persons.[6]

During the 1890s, AMO physicians steadily gave more attention to strategies to curtail propagation by defective persons. Partly as a result of the celebrated study, *The Jukes* (1877), and similar works, alarm continued to grow over the allegedly high fertility of the feeble-minded. In 1890 Dr. R. A. Mott, director of the Minnesota Institution for Defectives, stated flatly that "the fertility of the feeble-minded is proverbial." This was the cornerstone of his argument that the state had a duty to incarcerate defective persons until they were past reproductive age.[7]

The 1890 census evoked much pessimism in AMO circles. Kerlin felt that the new data indicated "a steady relative increase in the proportion of idiocy and imbecility to the general population." By the mid-1890s there was a growing conviction among the medical experts that the ineluctable power of heredity, the problem of hyperfecundity, and the growing difficulty of obtaining needed funds required that the institutions direct their efforts to prevent propagation by any defective person in the society. In 1895, Dr. A. W. Wilmarth, president of the Association for Mental Deficiency (as the AMO had been renamed), observed that it would soon be necessary to prevent *all* marriages by feeble-minded persons and to isolate all idiots.[8]

The intensity of these concerns was to no small degree a result of cost calculations that had been made by Dugdale when he studied the Jukes. Extrapolating from 834 of the individuals whom he had investigated, Dugdale concluded that there had been 1,200 family members during the last five generations. Using this number, he guessed the number of paupers, criminals, habitual thieves, prostitutes, syphilitics, and illegitimate children. He then estimated the costs to society that these persons had generated during their lives (table 1). Of interest is the emphasis he placed on the social costs of prostitution.

Dugdale concluded that the Jukes had cost the state

> over a million and a quarter dollars of loss in 75 years, caused by a single family 1,200 strong, without reckoning the cash paid for whiskey, or taking into account the entailment of pauperism and crime of the survivors in succeeding generations, and the incurable disease, idiocy, and insanity growing out of this debauchery, and reaching further than we can calculate. It is getting to be time to ask, do our courts, our laws, our alms-houses and our jails deal with the question presented?[9]

The Jukes saga quickly rooted in American soil. The *Atlantic Monthly* and the *Westminster Review* were among the popular journals that carried stories about the problem of "criminal" families. The story influenced professional circles as well. In 1884 Dr. Kerlin, speaking before the Eleventh National Conference of Charities and Reforms, noted that "Max and Ada Juke rarely fail of an introduction in these Conferences."[10] The next year, speaking at the Twelfth National Conference of Charities and Reforms, Kerlin used the Jukes story to argue that any legislature that refused to support its asylums was making a foolish error.[11] Three years later, speaking before the same group, the Reverend Oscar McCulloch, an en-

Table 1   Dugdale's Estimate of the Costs of the Jukes to New York by 1877

		Cost
Total number of persons	1,200	—
Number of pauperized adults	280	—
Cost of almshouse relief	—	15,000
Cost of outdoor relief	—	32,250
Number of criminals and offenders	140	—
Years of imprisonment	140	—
Cost of maintenance @ $200 a year	—	28,000
Number of arrests and trials, $100 each	—	25,000
Number of habitual thieves, convicted and unconvicted	60	—
Number of years of depredation, at 12 years each	720	—
Cost of depredation, $120 a year	—	86,400
Number of lives sacrificed by murder	7	—
Value, at $1,200 each	—	8,400
Number of common prostitutes	50	—
Average number of years of debauch	15	—
Total number of years of debauch	750	—
Cost of maintaining each per year	300	—
Cost of maintenance	—	225,000
Number of women specifically diseased	40	—
Average number of men each woman contaminates with permanent disease	10	—
Total number of men contaminated	400	—
Number of wives contaminated by above men	40	—
Total number of persons contaminated	440	—
Cost of drugs and medical treatment during rest of life, at $200 each	—	88,000
Average loss of wages caused by disease during rest of life, years	3	—
Total years of wages lost by 400 men	1,200	—
Loss at $500 a year	—	600,000
Average number of years withdrawn from productive industry by each courtesan	10	—
Total number of years lost by 50 courtesans	500	—
Value estimated at $125 a year	—	62,500
Aggregate curtailment of life of 490 adults, equivalent to 50 mature individuals	50	—
Cash cost, each life at $1,200	—	60,000
Aggregate of children who died prematurely	300	—
Average years of life of each child	2	—
Cash cost, each child at $50	—	15,000
Number of prosecutions in bastardy	30	—
Average cost of each case, $100	—	3,000

Table 1 *(continued)*

Cost of property destroyed, blackmail, brawls	—	20,000
Average capital employed in houses, stock, furniture, etc., for brothers	—	6,000
Compound interest for 26 years at 6 percent	—	18,000
Charity distributed by church	—	10,000
Charity obtained by begging	—	5,450
Total		$1,308,000

Source: Dugdale's table as it originally appeared in *The Jukes*, pp. 69-70.

ergetic social reformer from Indiana, delivered an account, "The Tribe of Ishmael: A Study in Social Degradation." His study of the "Ishmaelites" supported the findings of other studies that the unfit were unusually fecund. According to McCulloch, over five generations three brothers had engendered 1,750 descendants, many of whom had led deviant lives. Although it had a veneer of science, the study, which contained no information on the fecundity of normal persons, hardly constituted a careful analysis of fertility of the feeble-minded.[12]

Work in other disciplines seemed to confirm the concerns raised by Dugdale, McCulloch, and their colleagues. For example, Henry M. Boies, the aforementioned criminologist, reported that between 1850 and 1890, while the population of the United States had increased 170 percent, the criminal population had increased 445 percent. He attributed the differential partly to the freeing of the slaves, to immigration, and to intemperance, but he expressed his most grave concern for the high fertility of the criminal "classes." Boies reported that in Pennsylvania between 1880 and 1890, the number of inmates in penal institutions had increased 50 percent more quickly than had the growth of the state's population. The number of known defectives and "sane" paupers also significantly outpaced the general rise in population. In a single decade, the cost of running state institutions to house degenerates had increased an alarming 35 percent.[13]

By the turn of the century, the financial burden of dealing with crime was a serious public concern. At the annual meeting of the National Prison Association in 1900, Eugene Smith, a distinguished New York lawyer, delivered a paper entitled "The Cost of Crime," in which he estimated the annual expense to be about $600,000,000. A decade later a physician reported that the Massachusetts Prison Association now estimated that the cost of responding to crime was larger than any other item in the state budget except public education.[14] This again seemed to confirm Dugdale's findings that the Jukes had cost the people of New York over $1,250,000.[15]

During the period 1890-1910 there was also much concern for protecting the racial integrity of the United States. Attention turned to the problem of restricting the immigration of "weaker" stocks. Beginning about 1905 there was a dramatic increase in the attention devoted by the popular press to this problem. The *Reader's Guide to Periodical Literature* listed 27 articles under the "eugenics" entry between 1905 and 1909. Interested readers were offered cross-references to "degeneration," "heredity," and "race decadence." During the next five-year period, 122 entries were listed under "eugenics," making it one of the most referenced subjects in the index. Clearly, the reading public was routinely being confronted with these issues. Not a few of the articles, such as "Race Suicide and Racial Stamina," "The Future of the Human Race," and "Our Defectives," were unquestionably alarmist in tone. They helped create a climate in which radical solutions could gain currency.

Charles B. Davenport and the Eugenics Record Office

The popularity of this new literary topic can be in part credited to the efforts of Charles Benedict Davenport. Born in Brooklyn in 1866, Davenport first studied engineering. But soon after taking a degree from Brooklyn Polytechnic Institute, he defied his father's wishes and went to Harvard to study biology. After twelve years in Cambridge, seven of them as a lowly instructor, he next spent five years (1899-1904) at the University of Chicago, rising to associate professor. It was during this period (1902-4) that Davenport convinced officials at the newly endowed Carnegie Institute of Washington to create the Station for Experimental Evolution at Cold Spring Harbor, a campaign that also brought him the directorship in 1904.[16]

Trained in both mathematics and natural history, the young, ambitious Davenport was perfectly poised to appreciate the historic implications of the rediscovery of Mendel's work in plant breeding. In November 1900 he completed a paper that analyzed the work of Correns and De Vries, two of the three Europeans who had begun to spread the gospel of Mendelism. By 1904 Davenport had broken completely with the Galtonian school of biometrics and was deeply involved with Mendelian experiments on "unit characters" like coat color in animals. Euphoric over what he perceived to be the elegant simplicity of Mendel's laws and convinced of their application to human heredity, Davenport moved quickly to study people rather than poultry or peas. In 1908 he published a paper on the inheritance of eye color and skin color in humans.[17] By this time Davenport was convinced that there should be a second institution at Cold Spring Harbor, independent of the Station for Experimental Evolution, that could devote itself exclusively to the study of human heredity.

The key task was to secure a financial patron for this new venture. As it had been in 1903 when the Carnegie Institute funded his new laboratory, luck was again at Davenport's side. In September 1909 E. H. Harriman, the railroad magnate, died, leaving his philanthropically minded wife an estate worth 70 million dollars. Davenport had taught genetics to their daughter, Mary, in the summer of 1906. Waiting discreetly for the first tidal wave of supplicants to subside, Davenport used his acquaintance with Mary to arrange a discussion with Mrs. Harriman about creating a Eugenics Record Office (ERO), an institution dedicated exclusively to the genetic improvement of mankind. Mrs. Harriman was fascinated with the possibility that major social problems could be solved by identifying and eliminating defective genes from the human gene pool. She agreed to pay for the necessary buildings and to fund the ERO for five years. True to her words, from 1910 to 1917 she gave almost $250,000, nearly 85 percent of its budget.[18] Davenport quickly assembled a team of researchers and developed a program to collect genetic histories of families that seemed to carry defective genes. Trained field workers, most of them young women, searched the files of prisons, almshouses, and hospitals to identify suspect individuals and then gathered pedigree data. Over the next two decades they amassed data on hundreds of thousands of persons. Davenport also hired several persons to prepare monographs on particularly illustrative families. Of the five major studies of "degenerate" families that were published just before World War I, Davenport and his colleagues wrote four.

In August 1912 Florence H. Danielson, a field worker whom Davenport had trained, and Davenport published *The Hill Folk: Report on a Rural Community of Hereditary Defectives*. It strongly suggested that defective persons were highly fertile. They argued that for paupers "early marriages are the rule," and that there inevitably followed a large family of children with "fairly robust, physical constitutions." As evidence that such families were social burdens, Davenport charted one marriage that had produced "at least eleven children of which seven were definitely feeble-minded."[19] Another ERO monograph, *The Nam Family: a Study in Cacogenics,* was based on field work conducted by Dr. Arthur H. Estabrook in 1911. In Estabrook's view: "The rural communities of 'degenerates' usually have this in common: an unusual lack of industry, retardation in school work, and a failure to observe the conventionalities in sex relationships. There is reason for concluding that the first and second traits are hereditary and are in a measure, the raison d'être of the foundation of such communities. The last may be, in large measure, due to the remoteness of the community from social influences."[20]

In the fall of 1911 Mrs. O. F. Lewis, the wife of the general secretary of the Prison Association of New York, discovered the notes from which Dugdale had written *The Jukes* in 1877. Since Dugdale had died many years earlier, she contacted the ERO and allowed Estabrook to use this material. Estabrook spent three years tracing members of the Jukes family (who were now scattered over fourteen states). He reported that although time and change had disrupted rural isolation and dispersed the family, wherever they settled the immigrants tended to marry persons like themselves. Eschewing Dugdale's cautious analysis of the relative contributions of heredity and environment, Estabrook and Davenport (who guided the research and wrote the preface) bluntly ascribed the more important role to the germ plasm. They found support in Weismann, the German biologist who had developed the theory of the continuity of the germ plasm, and Mendel. If mental defect was programmed into the germ plasm and obeyed Mendel's laws, then the offspring of certain unfortunate matings were clearly doomed.[21]

The Kallikak Family

Influential as the ERO family studies were, another book, *The Kallikak Family*, published by Henry Herbert Goddard in 1912, was the work that really captured the contemporary imagination and greatly reinforced belief in the heritability of feeble-mindedness.[22]

Goddard grew up in Maine in a family of Quakers. After graduating from Haverford in 1887, he taught for a short time at the infant University of Southern California. Among the most esoteric of trivia is the fact that this future giant in the field of psychology was the first football coach at USC. Goddard returned to the East in the early nineties to pursue doctoral studies with G. Stanley Hall at Clark University. After earning a Ph.D. in 1899, he spent six years teaching in Westchester, New York. In 1906 Edward J. Johnstone, director of the Vineland Training School in New Jersey, who had convinced Samuel Fels, a wealthy Philadelphia soap merchant, to support studies of the etiology of feeble-mindedness, recruited Goddard to start a research department. Goddard spent his first eighteen months at Vineland engaged in detailed observations of and trying to develop new ways to test feeble-minded children. He hoped to discover factors that would identify those who were educable. After a year and a half without success, he went to France to learn what innovative psychologists there were doing. In Paris he met Théodore Simon and Alfred Binet and learned how they were using new testing methods to rank intelligence in children. In 1908 Goddard brought the first I.Q. tests to the United States, documents that Elizabeth Kite, his research assistant, translated.[23]

Goddard's trip changed the approach to measuring intelligence in the United States. Under Davenport's influence he had already studied the families of persons institutionalized at Vineland, and had been very surprised to discover so much mental defectiveness in relatives.[24] Now armed with a tool for investigating the intellectual capacity of the Vineland pupils, Goddard began to explore the inheritance of mental defects by studying test results within and between families. By 1910 he and Elizabeth Kite were deeply involved in a study of 327 families that would eventually form the basis for a massive book, *Feeble-Mindedness: Its Causes and Consequences.* [25] While engaged in that work, Kite and Goddard noticed that they had acquired unusually full and reliable material on a family that had lived in the Piney Woods of south central New Jersey for more than 150 years, a span of six generations. There was something almost irresistible about the Kallikak story.

Martin Kallikak, the progenitor of the line that eventually produced Deborah, a Vineland resident, came from a successful Quaker family. At the outbreak of the Revolutionary War he had broken with his nonviolent family to fight against England. During his army days he fathered an illegitimate son with a girl who lived in a Piney Woods settlement. After the war, he settled on a large, productive farm less than twenty miles away, married a respectable young woman, and started a legitimate line that prospered in central New Jersey. The family became eminent, producing judges and professors, and even publishing its own genealogy. Kite and Goddard could compare the two lines, one mothered by a Piney Woods dullard, the other by an intelligent, industrious Quaker maid.[26]

The manner in which Goddard described the two families shows that he thought the study offered important insight into the relative roles of heredity and environment as causes of feeble-mindedness:

> We thus have two series from two different mothers, but the same father. These extend for six generations. Both lines live out their lives in practically the same region and in the same environment, except in so far as they themselves, because of their different characters, changed that environment. Indeed, so close are they that in one case, a defective man on the bad side of the family was found in the employ of a family on the normal side and, although they are of the same name, neither suspects any relationship.
>
> We thus have a natural experiment of remarkable value to the sociologist and the student of heredity. That we are dealing with a problem of true

heredity, no one can doubt, for, although of the descendants of Martin Kallikak Jr. many married into feeble-minded families and thus brought in more
bad blood, yet Martin Jr. himself married a normal woman, thus demonstrat-
ing that the defect is transmitted through the mother, at least in this generation. Moreover, the Kallikak family traits appear continually even down to
the present generation, and there are many qualities that are alike in the good
and the bad families, thus showing the strength and persistence of the ancestral stock.[27]

Goddard's work supported two ideas that were central to those who
opposed propagation by the unfit. First, he seemed to have proved that
feeble-mindedness could be transmitted in a dominant fashion. Second, the
impressively large cohort of children born to each generation of the Piney
Woods line (one Millard Kallikak sired eighteen children by two wives)
when compared to the four- and five-child families of the "eminent" Kallikaks showed that the feeble-minded were highly fertile.

Written in clear language, embellished with photographs that compared attractive Deborah to her moronic and sinister-looking, noninstitutionalized relatives, and relatively short, *The Kallikak Family* hit home with
the public. Macmillan reprinted the book in 1913, 1914, 1916, and 1919,
and it won Goddard a measure of fame. Not until 1981, when it was
discovered that the photographs had been altered to make Deborah appear
better groomed and more attractive than her relatives, was the integrity of
the entire investigation cast in doubt.[28] But in 1912 one could not read the
book without asking whether the future of the society demanded that
propagation by the unfit be prevented.

Eugenics and Restrictive Legislation

One of the major social problems in America at the turn of the century
was caused by the dramatic influx of immigrants. Many of the newcomers
struck hard ground rather than fertile soil. From the 1870s forward, a
significant fraction of the persons in the almshouses in Boston, New York,
and Philadelphia were foreigners. As the years passed and the waves of
immigration swelled, so inevitably did the number of paupers who cla-
mored to sit at the dinner tables of the poorhouses. The cost of feeding the
poor was, however, a minor problem compared to mollifying the anger
among organized, native-born laborers caused by the arrival of tens of
thousands of men and women willing to work at a starvation wage scale.
Although the great unions were committed in principle to the international
alliance of workers, they yielded to the rank and file who had lost jobs to
strangely dressed men speaking mysterious tongues. The Knights of Labor

came out in favor of restricting immigration in 1892, and the more influential American Federation of Labor followed in 1894 when it officially endorsed a literacy test as a condition of entry into the United States. In many states American workers lobbied successfully to prevent aliens from competing with them. In 1894 and 1895 New York and Pennsylvania excluded the newcomers from jobs in state and local public works.[29]

Naturally, those who felt threatened by the rising tide of immigration sought arguments to legitimize their opposition. As early as the 1840s (which saw the first and smallest of four great waves of immigration), there were those who argued that the aliens were weakening rather than strengthening the nation. During the 1890s and in the first years of the new century, when immigration exceeded the wildest predictions—rising from 225,000 in 1898 to 1,300,000 in 1907—restrictionists seized on the eugenic argument.

To a eugenicist, who saw the world through glasses tinted with a hereditarian shade, there were much data to suggest that a disproportionally large number of immigrants arose from defective stock. In 1848 the Charity Hospital of New Orleans admitted 11,945 patients, of whom 10,280 were foreigners. In 1854 Jeremiah Clemens, a United States senator from Alabama, reported that during the prior year the New York Alms House had cared for 2,198 persons, of whom 1,633 were aliens. Similarly, over the prior six years the New York Lunatic Asylum had admitted 779 native-born Americans and 2,381 foreigners.[30]

There was little federal legislation on immigration until 1875. But from then until 1924, immigration bills were almost constantly before the Congress. The complicated record of these many bills indicates a steady increase in the classes of persons proposed for exclusion from the nation's shores. Concerns for cost and for protecting "American" racial integrity were the two cornerstones for this policy. A law enacted in 1875 prohibited the importation of women for prostitution and forbade entry by ex-convicts. Neutral on its face, the law was intended to deal with problems raised in California by the huge influx of coolie laborers. As implemented, it sharply reduced the entry of Oriental women and, therefore, the chance for Oriental men to find wives. This in turn encouraged the men to return to China. In 1882 a new law for the first time excluded lunatics, idiots, and persons likely to be a public charge. An important provision made shipowners bear the cost of returning excluded aliens, a rule intended to enhance screening at the European ports.[31]

According to the Select Committee to Inquire into the Importation of Contract Laborers, Convicts, and Paupers, which filed its report in 1889, measures to exclude "inadequate" persons were not enforced. That study helped generate a tougher law that was enacted in 1891. Besides Chinese laborers, it excluded idiots, insane persons, and persons convicted of crimes of moral turpitude. By 1901 President Theodore Roosevelt, an outspoken nativist, was urging even more restrictive laws. An ardent Social Darwinist who abhorred the flood of "weaker" stocks into his nation, Roosevelt wanted not merely to exclude defectives but to screen carefully for "intelligent capacity to appreciate American institutions." He supported a proposal to condition entry into the United States upon proof of literacy in some language, an idea that was hotly debated. Congress once did pass a literacy law, but President Cleveland vetoed it.[32]

In 1903 a new immigration law was enacted, which forbade the admission of epileptics and persons who had ever been insane, as well as any person afflicted with one of a host of medical problems. In 1907, at the height of a tidal wave of aliens, the exclusion was enlarged to block the entry of imbeciles, feeble-minded persons, and individuals suffering from tuberculosis. Shipowners who carried such persons could be fined one hundred dollars per person. The steady extension of the list of excluded persons dovetailed well with prevalent theories as to the hereditary nature of these kinds of defects, including the tendency to contract tuberculosis.[33]

The most vigorously articulated eugenic arguments against immigration were voiced by the Immigration Restriction League (IRL). The IRL was started in Boston in 1894 by five young Harvard graduates who were concerned by the social cost to their city generated by the many poor Irish who had recently arrived. Throughout its history the IRL was small, but rich and influential. It had the ear of Senator Henry Cabot Lodge, lobbied effectively in Washington, and mailed its literature directly to five hundred daily newspapers. It led the struggle in favor of a literacy test. The IRL was a forerunner of the more strident voices that would vigorously attack the nation's relatively liberal immigration policy before and after World War I. Its arguments about the inferiority of Italians were precursors of the blatantly racist jeremiads later made by eugenicists like Madison Grant.[34]

The economic problems caused by the influx of immigrants in the 1890s (a decade torn by labor unrest and an economic depression) and fears for the impact that these millions of strangers would have on America's racial stock gave a sense of urgency to the problem of the rapidly increasing number of native-born dependent persons. However, another major demographic change also fostered concern: the rising level of miscegenation between blacks and whites.

Although there was unquestionably extensive miscegenation throughout the nation's history, in the decades after the Civil War there arose deep concern, especially among southern whites, that it was increasing at a dangerous pace.[35] According to one authority, between 1890 and 1910 the colored population increased by 81 percent, while the Negro population increased by only 23 percent. Another writer asserted that between 1859 and 1910 the mulatto population increased 500 percent.[36] During the last quarter of the nineteenth century the legal restrictions on miscegenation were tightened. The usual way in which this was accomplished was to enact a broader definition of "Negro." Between 1875 and 1924, many states amended their statutes to make it illegal for a white person to marry any person who had "one-sixteenth or more Negro blood." Some eventually defined as such any person in whom it could be shown that there was a single drop of Negro blood.[37]

During this era there was also a flood of new laws prohibiting marriages between whites and Orientals. Of the ten states that enacted such laws, nine were located west of the Mississippi River. This was a calculated response to the huge influx of Chinese laborers who were imported to build the transcontinental railroads. "You can work here, but you can't stay on after the job is done," seemed to be the message of the laws. There were few legal challenges to the statutes. In those that did occur, the courts were unanimous in upholding their constitutionality. In Indiana (1871), Alabama (1877), Texas (1877), Arkansas (1875), and Louisiana (1907), courts upheld the power of the state to prohibit interracial marriage.[38] People who approved of these laws were likely to support analogous measures intended to protect the nation from other threats, including childbearing by the feeble-minded.

During the 1880s, as the number of persons housed in state-supported facilities continued to grow rapidly, concern about the fecundity of the feeble-minded increased. New laws that forbade children between the ages of two and sixteen to reside in almshouses increased the length of the waiting lists for admission to the schools for the feeble-minded. There was also a growing certainty that many retarded persons had inherited their defects. In 1886 Dr. J. C. Carson, who worked at the Newark facility, compiled "an hereditary analysis of applications for admission." He gloomily concluded that the data left little doubt that feeble-mindedness ran strongly in families. He was sure that as he gathered more data, "the hereditary coloring would appear still darker."[39]

By 1890 the policy of lifetime segregation of feeble-minded women was widely accepted by officials who only fifteen years earlier had opposed custodial care. Dr. R. A. Mott, director of the Minnesota Institute for Defectives, acknowledged that his goal was "to keep the persons entrusted to our care until they are past the reproducing age, and reduce hereditary epilepsy and imbecility within the lines of our republic to a minimum."[40] The 1890 census, which revealed yet another dramatic increase in the number of idiots and imbeciles, reinforced arguments favoring strict segregation of retarded women. By 1895 experts were even advocating measures that would reach the vast majority of feeble-minded persons who were *not* institutionalized. As one physician perceived it, the problem had reached such alarming proportions that it was inevitable that "before another generation comes about means will be taken to prevent the marriage of feeble-minded persons, and idiotic persons will be kept apart."[41]

The policy of segregating feeble-minded women to reduce their risk of pregnancy was soon widely accepted. However, given the small percentage of all feeble-minded persons who were housed in institutions and the unlikelihood of securing funds to accommodate more than a fraction of such persons at state expense, it was not surprising that other solutions would emerge. Perhaps most ardent was a congressman who, convinced of the hereditary factors in crime, proposed establishing a penal colony in Alaska to which all the nation's habitual criminals would be exiled.[42]

In 1895 Connecticut became the first state to prohibit the marriage of defective persons. Except when the woman was forty-five or older, parties to a marriage, either of whom was "epileptic, imbecile or feeble-minded" could be imprisoned for up to three years. The ban also extended to unmarried persons. Here the law had a broader reach. In addition to other constraints, any "pauper" who "carnally" knew any female under the age of forty-five was also subject to a three-year prison term. Marriage restriction laws enjoyed a certain vogue for almost twenty years. By 1913 they had been enacted in twenty-four states, the District of Columbia, and Puerto Rico. The vast majority forbade marriages of people who were epileptic, idiot or imbecile, insane, or feeble-minded. A few states forbade the marriage of paupers, drunkards, or persons with "physical incapacity." Washington had perhaps the nation's most eugenic law. That state prohibited marriage by epileptics, idiots or imbeciles, the feeble-minded, habitual criminals, drunkards, the insane, persons with advanced tuberculosis, and persons with venereal disease. Paupers were spared.[43]

In 1913 Davenport analyzed the statutes from a eugenic prospective. While he applauded the intent of the laws and thought that they were targeted at appropriate classes, Davenport doubted whether there was biological evidence to justify prohibiting the marriage of a defective person with a person free from neuropathic taint. Applying an overly simplified Mendelian analysis, he thought that children of such a couple would be "mentally normal—or affected, at most, with a slight nervousness." His analysis of twelve marriages, each between a normal person and a neuropathic individual, showed that of fifty children, all were "normal except for one quarrelsome, one alcoholic and one nervous." Davenport concluded that the marriage restriction laws would not achieve their goal. As to the feeble-minded, whom he believed had "weak sex control," restrictive legislation had no deterrent force. He characterized laws forbidding the marriage of epileptics as unenforceable and, for those persons affected with milder forms of the disease, unfair. Because he thought that most cases of insanity usually developed in mid-adulthood, Davenport thought that marriage prohibitions would have little impact on this problem. The only disorder for which he felt that restrictive marriage laws made good sense was Huntington's chorea, a late onset neurological disorder that was first described on Long Island and that he had studied.[44] In Davenport's words: "the proper action in the case of imbeciles or the gross epileptics who wish to marry is not to decline to give them a marriage license, but to place them in an institution under state care during at least the entire reproductive period. No cheap device of a law against marriage will take the place of compulsory segregation of gross defectives."[45]

It does not appear that marriage restriction laws were ever strongly enforced. For example, in 1905 the Supreme Court of Connecticut, in ruling that a woman whose husband had concealed that he suffered from epilepsy could file for divorce on the grounds of fraud, noted that its ten-year-old law had never before been invoked. The court's opinion provides an extraordinary insight into the view commonly held of epilepsy in that era: "That epilepsy is a disease of a peculiarly serious and revolting character, tending to weaken mental force, and often descending from parent to child, or entailing upon the offspring of the sufferer some other grave form of nervous malady, is a matter of common knowledge, of which courts will take judicial notice."[46]

Laws that prohibited the marriage of the feeble-minded, the insane, and persons suffering from epilepsy were enacted in a climate of pseudoscientific certainty. In eugenic circles the overriding importance of heredity was viewed as an established fact. As the more cautious and less politically active scientists and physicians did not speak out, the pro-eugenic evidence seemed more impressive than it really was. For example, in 1911 A. J. Rosanoff, a physician-eugenicist, reported that his studies of the insane, many of whom were said also to be afflicted with epilepsy, indicated that one-fourth of the *entire population* carried germ cells defective in neuropathic strength.[47] A few years later, at the height of legislative interest in restricting dysgenic marriages, such scientific treatises provided proponents with a ready source of support.

Given this climate, it was hardly surprising that some persons would embrace radical solutions to deal with the rising crime rate, rampant prostitution, and other social problems. Several legislatures seriously considered and two nearly adopted laws providing for the castration of persons convicted of rape or murder. The legislative history of bills to castrate persons convicted of certain crimes dates at least to 1855. In that year the territorial legislature of Kansas enacted a law permitting the castration of any "negro or mulatto" who was convicted of rape, attempted rape, or kidnapping any white woman. It was later amended to provide for the castration of rapists regardless of color. In 1907 a bill was introduced in the Texas legislature making rape, assault with intent to commit rape, and incest punishable by castration. The bill was passed by the House with only two dissenting votes, but died in the Senate.[48]

Perhaps the most colorful of the early advocates of castration was Gideon Lincecum, a self-taught Texas physician. In 1848 Lincecum gave up a lucrative practice in Columbus, Mississippi, and moved to Texas. There he reestablished his practice, but devoted much of his life to studying natural history and pursuing social causes. In 1849 he performed autopsies on three persons who had been executed, an experience that led him to develop the curious thesis that emasculation was a more humane way than hanging to deal with convicted murderers. By 1854 Dr. Lincecum was so convinced of his views that he prepared an essay that he sent to more than six hundred lawmakers, newspaper editors, and physicians. In his view, the rising crime rate proved that current penal law had failed. This was because "it is the animal and not the intellectual portion of our organic structure that commits crime and does violence." Simply put, the cause of crime was lust.

He argued that the threat of castration would deter criminal activity. He also believed that it would convert the callous criminal to a compassionate citizen. As proof he described a

> vicious, disobedient, indolent, drunken Negro who was in the habit of committing rape on the wenches of his own race, and whom the neighbors had threatened to shoot. After discovering that he had impregnated an idiot white girl, three men went into the field where he was at work and castrated him. Less than two years later I heard his mistress say that he had become a model servant who never slept, until every young and tender thing about the place was fully provided for; lamb, pig, or young chicken—all received his protecting care.[49]

Lincecum was ridiculed by the press, but a few years later in 1864 a jury in Belton, Texas, convicted a Negro of rape and recommended castration, a sentence that was carried out. This may be the only legal castration in the country's history.

Arguments favoring eugenic and punitive castration were not uncommon in the 1890s. A major controversy over castration occurred in 1894 when Dr. Hoyt Pilcher, superintendent of the Asylum for Idiots and Feeble-minded Youths in Winfield, Kansas, disclosed that he had castrated fourteen girls and forty-four boys. Most were adolescents known by Dr. Pilcher to be chronic masturbators, a practice that he believed would exacerbate their retardation. When a local newspaper broke the story about the Winfield castrations, a brouhaha ensued that cost Dr. Pilcher his job. But an editorial in the *Kansas Medical Journal* strongly favored the salubrious effects of castration and asserted that "these operations are occurring constantly."[50]

Castration was too brutal to provide a socially acceptable solution to curbing the fecundity of the feeble-minded. In the early 1900s, however, it provided a foil against which sterilization seemed humane and politically more palatable.

3 · The Surgical Solution

> If it were possible to eliminate all habitual criminals from the possibility of having children, there would soon be a very marked decrease in this class, and naturally, also a consequent decrease in the number of criminals from contact.
>
> —A. J. Ochsner, "Surgical Treatment of Habitual Criminals," *Journal of the American Medical Association*, April 22, 1899

> "Defendant Is Sterilized to Get Lesser Sentence."
>
> —*New York Times*, July 22, 1986

The earliest American case report of a vasectomy, published by A. J. Ochsner, chief surgeon at St. Mary's Hospital and Augustana Hospital in Chicago, described two patients who had consulted him because of prostate problems in the summer of 1897. The first patient, who had been bothered by prostatitis for three months, was much improved two weeks after the vasectomy. At follow-up twenty months later, the patient reported that his "sexual power," which had been somewhat impaired before the operation, was "as good as at any time during his life." Ochsner noted similar positive results with his second patient.

Ochsner's report was unusual for two different reasons. First, there is no physiologic basis for supposing that severing the vas deferens should ameliorate prostatic hypertrophy, cure prostatitis, or increase sexual vigor. One is forced to attribute the improvements in the patients to chance or to a placebo effect from the surgery. Second, the young surgeon chose to characterize the medical implications of his technical advance in a most unconventional manner. Consider the paper's title: "Surgical Treatment of Habitual Criminals." In his discussion Ochsner asserted that "it has been demonstrated beyond a doubt that a very large proportion of all criminals, degenerates, and perverts have come from parents similarly afflicted. It has also been shown, especially by Lombroso, that there are certain inherited anatomic defects which characterize criminals, so that there are undoubtedly born criminals."[1]

He then asserted that "if it were possible to eliminate all habitual criminals from the possibility of having children, there would soon be a very marked decrease in this class." Dr. Ochsner argued that the vasectomy offered a socially acceptable method of doing away with hereditary criminals from the "father's side," and that the same treatment "could reasonably be suggested for chronic inebriates, imbeciles, perverts and paupers." In a page of printed text he articulated a deceptively simple solution for stopping the rising tide of "racial degeneracy" that then so troubled America.

Ochsner performed his first vasectomy in 1897, an era when urologists were searching for a surgical treatment of prostatic hypertrophy. During the 1880s, some surgeons had castrated men with the most severe symptoms. But this operation was not curative, and it was nearly as dangerous for the surgeon as for the patient: at least one irate individual murdered the physician who had therapeutically castrated him. By 1890 a Philadelphia surgeon, Dr. J. Ewing Mears, favored the somewhat less mutilating therapy of ligating the spermatic cord. This physiologic castration (the operation destroyed the blood supply to the testicles) may have suggested the idea of vasectomy.[2]

Ochsner's paper on vasectomy was his only published contribution to the problem of "hereditary degeneracy." In 1900 he was appointed professor of clinical surgery at the University of Illinois, a post he held until just prior to his death in 1926. During his rich career he published four books, including a text on thyroid surgery, and served as president of the American College of Surgeons.[3] Although he did not champion eugenic sterilization, he may have influenced several prominent Midwestern surgeons who did.

On March 8, 1902, one of them, Dr. Harry C. Sharp, surgeon for the Indiana Reformatory, published the second major medical article that favored eugenic sterilization. Entitled "The Severing of the Vasa Deferentia and Its Relation to the Neuropsychopathic Constitution," it was virtually a manifesto for a sterilization movement. Sharp first marshaled proof of the existence of "laws" of heredity. Although he mentioned Galton and cited French psychologist Théodule Ribot, he was apparently not yet aware of Mendel's work, soon to be used by eugenicists such as Davenport to argue that the various expressions of neuropathic weakness (criminality, pauperism, etc.) were transmitted in a simple, particulate manner.[4] Sharp was less concerned with the etiology of defective germ plasm than he was with its rapidly increasing burden. Reviewing U.S. census data he noted that

> in 1850 there were 6,737 criminals in the United States, or one to each 3,442 of the population; while in 1890 the penal population is shown to be 83,329 or one to each 957 of the population. This is of the criminal alone. If all

dependents were considered, such as inhabit public and private insane hospitals, almshouses and institutes for the feeble-minded we should find the proportion to be in the neighborhood of one to three hundred of the population.

Sharp found this most alarming and called for "a most heroic method of treatment," one that he had initiated.[5]

Dr. Sharp reported that in an effort to prevent the birth of criminals he had personally severed the vasa deferentia of forty-two prison inmates whose ages ranged from seventeen to twenty-five. After vasectomy, he wrote, the patients "feel that they are stronger, sleep better, their memory improves, the will becomes stronger, and they do better in school." Convinced of his findings, he urged his fellow physicians to prevail upon legislatures to empower the directors of state institutions "to render every male sterile who passes its portals, whether it be almshouse, insane asylum, institute for the feeble-minded, reformatory or prison."

Sharp's paper is important for three reasons. It made the first florid exaggerations of the benefits flowing from vasectomy, assertions that would become common as more physicians became advocates of eugenic sterilization. Second, it made the first call for a lobbying effort by physicians in favor of sterilization laws. Third, it documented the world's first episode of mass sterilization (performed without court approval or patient consent) of institutionalized persons.

During the next few years the number of physicians advocating eugenic sterilization mushroomed, and many published pro-sterilization articles. A typical example is the first such piece to appear in a California medical journal. The author, Dr. R. C. Ellinwood, described a teen-age boy who became maniacal "under sexual excitement." According to Ellinwood, after undergoing a vasectomy the boy's attacks of rage disappeared. He became "quite industrious, ambitious to work and happy in following his trade."[6]

As physicians became familiar with this simple operation, a few began to lobby vociferously in favor of mass sterilization of defective men. At the 1905 meeting of the Association of American Institutions for the Feeble-Minded, held in New Jersey, Dr. S. D. Risley drew a gloomy picture of an America threatened by hordes of defectives. He was convinced that "not only are vast numbers of hereditary paupers, imbeciles, inebriates, and criminals being born annually in our midst to swell the number of these degenerates, but they are entering through the too widely open door of our immigration system." As Risley saw it, the problem was growing exponentially. He believed that "the child of the feeble-minded parent or of the criminal and the inebriate begins his vicious life not only earlier, but pursues it with a momentum not equaled by the parent." He was also convinced that masturbation exacerbated the underlying defects with which these people were burdened, aggravating their tendency to "epilepsy and other deranged mental states and other nervous disorders of ill-defined types." Vasectomy was the only solution to lift them from the "slough of degeneration."

Volleying an early round in the sterilization campaign, Risley sharply criticized the governor of Pennsylvania for vetoing a sterilization bill earlier that year. Describing the veto message as a striking example of the "psychologic tyranny of prejudice," Risley argued that it was imperative that physicians educate lawyers on these matters. Publication of his plea by the *Journal of Psycho-Asthenics,* the only English language periodical devoted exclusively to problems of caring for the feeble-minded, permitted it to reach an important professional audience.[7]

The Beginnings of Sterilization Legislation

The year 1907 was a critical moment in the history of eugenic sterilization. On April 9, 1907, about one month after two-thirds of the members of both houses had voted favorably, J. Frank Hanly, governor of Indiana, signed a law authorizing the compulsory sterilization of any confirmed criminal, idiot, rapist, or imbecile in a state institution whose condition had been determined to be "unimprovable" by an appointed panel of physicians.[8] The enactment of the first state law emboldened other legislatures to consider this controversial subject.

Dr. Sharp, who played a key role in lobbying for the Indiana law, quickly emerged as a national figure in the sterilization debate. Speaking in Chicago at the annual meeting of the National Prison Association (NPA), he reported that he had performed 223 operations on prisoners without a single complication. His follow-up studies indicated that both the physical and the mental condition of the patients had improved. In Sharp's mind there was a clear duty "to the future of our race and our nation, to see that the defective and diseased do not multiply."[9]

His remarks elicited generally favorable comment. For example, the superintendent of a leper colony in Cuba stated that he would change his current plan to sterilize lepers by radiation to the use of the vasectomy. An Ohio state official asserted that he hoped soon to obtain a law like Indiana's. Two delegates did express concern about the constitutionality of the Indiana law, but the NPA Standing Committee on Criminal Law Reform soon approved the new statute. A day later Dr. Sharp was elected president of the Physicians' Association of the NPA. Sometime during his year as president, Sharp privately published a pamphlet, *Vasectomy,* intended for use as a lobbying aid by proponents of sterilization bills. On the inside cover was affixed a postcard that readers could tear out, sign, and mail to their state representatives to show support for such a bill.

On August 12, 1909, Connecticut became the second state to adopt a law modeled on the Indiana plan. With the enactment of sterilization laws in Indiana and Connecticut, and the efforts of the indefatigable Dr. Sharp, interest within the medical profession in mass sterilization increased rapidly.

Early discussion of eugenic sterilization focused largely on men. Ochsner had considered the problem of the female criminal, but noted that "nature usually protects the community against the likelihood of (their) offspring, because a very large proportion of these individuals acquire a specific endometritis and salpingitis." His observation that prostitutes were often infertile because of chronic venereal infections was no doubt correct. Although he considered cutting the Fallopian tubes as a counterpart to eugenic vasectomy, he (correctly) judged it too dangerous. Despite occasional attempts in the United States as early as 1880, the salpingectomy was really developed by M. Madlener, a German surgeon. Between 1910 and 1920 he sterilized eighty-nine women with only three postoperative deaths, an excellent result for that era.[10] For Ochsner, Sharp, and other American physicians who were concerned about jails bursting with male prisoners, the problem of defective female germ plasm was of secondary importance. Given the immediacy of the (male) criminal problem, the epidemic of female sterility among the "degenerate" classes, and the vast difference in cost and morbidity between the vasectomy and salpingectomy, the focus on males made sense.

On December 13, 1907, Dr. William T. Belfield became the first surgeon of national academic reputation to speak in favor of mass eugenic sterilization. At the time, Belfield (who has been credited with performing the first suprapubic prostatectomy in 1886) was at the pinnacle of his career as professor of surgery at Rush Medical College. He had long been interested in forensic medicine and in 1903 had contributed a chapter on the microscopic examination of hairs to a textbook of legal medicine.[11] At a joint meeting of the Physicians' Club and the Law Club of Chicago, Dr. Belfield read a paper entitled "Race Suicide for Social Parasites," which was later abstracted in the *Journal of the American Medical Association.* Belfield noted that between 1881 and 1906 there had been a fourfold rise in the national homicide rate, and that the murder rate in Chicago was thirty-three times higher than in London. Convinced that the United States was being overrun by habitual criminals, Belfield viewed involuntary sterilization as the only solution. Praising the Indiana law, Belfield urged adoption of a similar program in Illinois.[12]

Advocacy within the medical profession for eugenic sterilization grew steadily; between 1909 and 1910, twenty-three papers on eugenic sterilization were listed in the *Index Medicus.* Every medical article published between 1899 and 1912 on eugenic sterilization favored this practice. These papers often had a most activist tone. Consider the article by Dr. Ewing Mears, the Philadelphia urologist, that appeared in the *Boston Medical and Surgical Journal.* The paper, "Asexualization as a Remedial Measure in the Relief of Certain Forms of Mental, Moral, and Physical Degeneration" (asexualization was here used to mean sterilization, not castration), urged surgery for stemming the tide of all kinds of "degeneracy," not just criminality. In this paper Mears mentioned that Dr. Thomas L. Stedman, an influential editor of the *Medical Record,* had provided him with a copy of Belfield's paper, indicating that sterilization advocates were coordinating their efforts. Mears bragged about pushing his advocacy of eugenic sterilization by writing to the directors of state institutions.[13]

In 1909 the *Journal of the American Medical Association* printed a speech read by Dr. Sharp to the Sixteenth Annual Session of the American Medical Association. Sharp asserted that between 1890 and 1908 the cost to Indiana of maintaining the institutions that housed various dependent persons had increased over 100 percent, and that the state's jail population had jumped from 600 in 1892 to 1,275 in 1908. After criticizing other proposals then circulating to limit propagation by the unfit (marriage restriction laws, segregation, and castration), Sharp reported the latest data on his sterilization campaign in Indiana. In ten years he had performed 456 vasectomies without a single serious complication. He claimed that after surgery his patients in the Jeffersonville Reformatory had a "more sunny disposition," were "brighter of intellect," and no longer masturbated excessively! Apparently abandoning an earlier concern about the surgical risks, Sharp proposed extending his program to the 300 girls in the state institution for the feeble-minded. As he saw it, "the only reason for detention is for the purpose of segregation as they have not the character to resist the importunities of unprincipled men."[14] Would not sterilization reduce the need for female institutionalization?

Sharp's remarks found a sympathetic audience. During the discussion Dr. Woods Hutchinson, a New York physician, reported that his analysis of family records at the Vineland State School had convinced him of the "enormous fecundity" of the feeble-minded. Dr. Charles Rosenwasser, vice-president of the Dependency and Crime Commission of New Jersey, noted that a study in Illinois had traced all the institutionalized delinquents to membership in fewer than 150 families. He disclosed his plan to introduce a bill into the New Jersey legislature proposing the compulsory sterilization of habitual criminals.[15] New Jersey did enact a sterilization law about eighteen months later.

Its passage may have been secured in part because of the efforts of Dr. David F. Weeks, a physician who had collaborated with Charles Davenport in the study of epilepsy. Weeks was chief physician at the New Jersey State Village for Epileptics, and given his large experience with defective persons, legislators probably relied heavily on his opinion. Once the New Jersey law was enacted, Dr. Weeks moved quickly to implement a sterilization program.[16]

Charles V. Carrington, surgeon at the Virginia State Penitentiary, was another physician willing to work as a lobbyist. Carrington asked his colleagues "to secure the passage of a law [a draft of which he had already written] by our next Legislature that will require the sterilization of certain classes of our criminals." As he saw it, a "good doctor has enormous weight in discussing such a subject with a thinking member of the Legislature." His efforts failed; Virginia did not enact a sterilization statute until 1924.[17]

In 1909, Dr. F. W. Hatch, secretary of the State Lunacy Commission in California, won a significant victory on behalf of eugenic sterilization. Convinced that most insanity was hereditary and incurable, he drafted a sterilization bill that was introduced by his friend, Senator W. F. Price. Perhaps the fears of "race-suicide" that had been engendered in many Californians by the heavy influx of Oriental immigrants had created a favorable climate for eugenic policy. The bill passed both houses with virtually no opposition and was signed by Governor James N. Gillett in June. Shortly after the statute was enacted, Dr. Hatch became general superintendent of state hospitals, a position that conferred upon him the power to implement the new law. From 1909 until his death in 1924, Hatch vigorously pursued a policy of mass sterilization of institutionalized persons, especially the insane. Under his direction the surgeons at ten state hospitals sterilized about three thousand persons.[18]

Of the many pro-sterilization papers published around 1910, two are of interest because of the prominence of their authors. In June of that year, Lewellys F. Barker, who succeeded the great William Osler as physician-in-chief at the Johns Hopkins Hospital, published a long article entitled "The Importance of the Eugenic Movement and Its Relation to Social Hygiene" in the *Journal of the American Medical Association*. As senior physician at the nation's leading medical school and one of the most influential voices in medicine, Barker's balanced discussion of human genetics and eugenics was surely influential. Although he did not endorse involuntary sterilization, his readers could conclude that Barker favored rational, enlightened eugenic practices. His paper indirectly legitimized eugenic thinking.[19]

On April 6, 1912, G. Frank Lydston, professor of genitourinary surgery at the University of Illinois, contributed a long article, "Sex Mutilations in Social Therapeutics," to the *New York Medical Journal*. [20] At fifty-five years of age and said to have the most lucrative surgical practice in Chicago, Dr. Lydston was recognized as one of the leading urologists in the Midwest. Besides publishing dozens of medical articles and a textbook on urology, he also had a keen interest in forensic medicine. He was a student of the Italian criminologist Cesare Lombroso, and for many years he held a professorship in criminal anthropology at the Kent College of Law.[21]

In December 1906 Dr. Lydston had published *Diseases of Society*, the first book in America to recommend sterilization of both sexes as a means of curtailing "social disease." This mammoth work, which purported to be a definitive investigation of the "vice and crime" problem in the United States, was obviously influenced by Lombroso. For example, the title page was flanked by a large drawing of a "skull of a Negro murderer." Lydston was most concerned with exploring the etiology of vice, so it was only in his final chapter, "Therapeutics of Social Disease," that he discussed sterilization. In his view:

> Sterilization, in both the male and female, has a wide range of application in the prevention of social disease. As already indicated, individuals whose physical or moral status is such as to insure the unfitness of their prospective progeny should be given the alternative of submitting to sterilization as the only condition upon which matrimony is legally permissible. Persons with a history of insanity, epileptics, dipsomaniacs, incurable syphilitics, certain persons who suffer from deformity or chronic disease, criminals, and persons with criminal records should not be permitted to marry upon any other conditions. Incurable criminals, epileptics, and the insane should invariably be submitted to the operation, irrespective of matrimony. Even the rare cases of reformed habitual criminals should be subjected to the operation, for the cure of their own criminal tendencies will not interfere with the transmission of those tendencies to their progeny.[22]

Lydston, an independent thinker and a perpetual critic of organized medicine, integrated his views on medicine and the social sciences to develop a somewhat idiosyncratic theory of sociology. He believed that the "criminal acts of the unfit really constitute diseases of the social body," and that the "medical doctor is the best social doctor as well." He unabashedly advocated radical social policies: castration of convicted rapists, thorough medical scrutiny of *all* applicants for a marriage license, with sterilization of unfit couples (consumptives, epileptics, the insane, incurable inebriates, and criminals) made a prerequisite to obtaining the license, and serious investigation of whether there should be a financial test of candidates for matrimony. He even advocated using a hermetically sealed apartment with a secret pipe for the admission of deadly gas "to kill promptly the convicted murderer and the driveling imbecile."[23]

The pro-eugenic stance of the *Texas Medical Journal* merits some mention. This little red monthly magazine was founded by Dr. F. E. Daniel, an Austin physician, in 1885 and edited and published by him until his death in May 1914. As early as 1893 Dr. Daniel journeyed to New York to read a paper advocating the castration of "insane criminals and sexual perverts" before the American Medico-Legal Society. In 1894 he thoroughly reported the scandal in Kansas that engulfed Dr. Pilcher when he admitted castrating retarded adolescents. Daniel reprinted an editorial from the *Kansas Medical Journal* defending Dr. Pilcher's actions.[24] In 1907 he came out strongly in favor of a bill providing that persons guilty of rape, attempted rape, or incest should be castrated, a measure that was approved by the Texas House but rejected by the Senate.[25]

In 1909 Dr. Daniel served as chairman of the Section on State Medicine and Public Hygiene of the Texas Medical Association. In his chairman's address, "Sterilization of Male Insane," he noted that the five Texas asylums were jammed with five thousand patients and predicted that by 1930 the state would need ten asylums and a huge budget. He urged the association's committee on legislation to ask passage of a sterilization law aimed at criminals and lunatics.[26]

Between 1910 and 1912, Dr. Daniel frequently published pro-sterilization articles by Dr. Henri G. Bogart, a physician from Brookville, Indiana. Bogart kept Texas physicians abreast of new laws favoring sterilization. In January 1913 Daniel launched a monthly column, "Department of Eugenics," which reported on the activities of the Texas State Society of Social Hygiene. With its headquarters in San Antonio, this society of fifteen eugenically minded physicians contributed a steady flow of manuscript material until Daniel's death. After that Mrs. Daniel, who did not share her husband's eugenic concerns, shifted the journal's focus to the problem of pellagra. Although Dr. Daniel never managed to secure a law for Texas, his tireless campaigning for sterilization earned him top marks as a physician activist.

The now-flaking pages of the medical journals and material in private archives provide good evidence to demonstrate that between 1900 and 1915 at least a few physicians were outspoken lobbyists for programs of involuntary sterilization to stop the spread of defective germ plasm. But what impact did these men have on the implementation of social policy? To help answer this question we must determine how many states passed sterilization laws during this era, and whether there was evidence that physicians lobbied on their behalf.

Between 1907 and 1913, legislatures in sixteen states passed sterilization bills, of which four (in Pennsylvania, Oregon, Vermont, and Nebraska) were vetoed by the governors. The twelve states that enacted sterilization laws were Indiana, Washington, California, Connecticut, Nevada, Iowa, New Jersey, New York, North Dakota, Michigan, Kansas, and Wisconsin. Indiana enacted the first law, and there the influence of Dr. Sharp cannot be ignored. In California, Connecticut, and New Jersey, prominent physicians, including persons who worked in the departments of public health, lobbied in favor of the sterilization bills that became law. From his office on the State Lunacy Commission, Dr. F. W. Hatch drafted the California bill and urged it upon friends in the legislature. In later years, one leader of the sterilization movement described Hatch as the key lobbyist on behalf of that bill.[27] In Connecticut, a number of prominent Hartford physicians wrote in favor of sterilization, but there is no clear evidence of their influence on the legislature. Dr. David F. Weeks, chief physician at the New Jersey State Village for Epileptics, was a vocal proponent of sterilization, and once the law was enacted in that state he quickly implemented it. However, evidence of his influence on the legislature is only circumstantial. Illinois, the home of several of the most prominent physicians who favored sterilization, never did adopt such a law.

In Pennsylvania and Oregon, physicians were the undisputed leaders of the pro-sterilization lobbying effort. Dr. Ewing Mears worked vigorously to secure passage of the 1905 bill in Pennsylvania and was outraged when the governor vetoed it. In Oregon, Dr. B. Owens-Adair led the pro-sterilization drive by publishing dozens of letters in the *Oregonian*. She was convinced that sterilization was the only social weapon available to combat the pollution of germ tissue by alcohol. She was of such stature that when the governor vetoed the bill, he wrote to her to explain his decision.[28]

The evidence indicates that a handful of activist physicians played an important role in securing passage of laws to permit the sterilization of "defective" persons. They educated their profession about the dimensions of a social problem and the existence of a new, relatively unobjectionable tool to fix it. One small problem was to explain the difference between castration and sterilization and to end the practice of calling both "asexualization." By 1909 many legislators apparently considered the vasectomy to be a tolerable surgical intervention.

Despite the enactment of twelve state laws permitting sterilization, the number of operations was modest. In the decade from 1907 to 1917 there were 1,422 sterilizations of institutionalized persons pursuant to state law.[29] Except for California, where more than half of all sterilizations took place, and Indiana, where Dr. Sharp acknowledged that he had sterilized several hundred more men than state records indicated, the laws were seldom utilized. Indeed, between 1913 and 1918 constitutional challenges were brought against seven of the laws, and *all* were declared invalid. With such a dismal record one might think that eugenic sterilization was a fad that would die out. In fact, the years before World War I were merely a prologue for a much more serious campaign that began soon after that great conflagration had burnt itself out.

4 · Sterilization Laws

Since this pioneer legislative act in the United States in behalf of eugenic and therapeutic human sterilization, our country has become the foremost champion and advocate of the cause in the world. Sixty-three different human sterilization acts have been enacted since the legal inception of this movement in the United States. Twenty-seven states may legally practice eugenic human sterilization in the Union today

—J. H. Landman, *Human Sterilization*, 1932

"Maryland Court OKs Involuntary Sterilization of Retarded Minors"

—*American Medical News*, August 6, 1982

In the years before World War I, advocates of eugenic sterilization were remarkably successful in securing state laws that targeted institutionalized persons, including prisoners, the feeble-minded, and the insane. In attempting to understand why state lawmakers passed sterilization bills in the early years of this century, one is hampered by a lack of legislative history. For example, the Connecticut State Library has no material in its legislative collection prior to 1911, two years after Connecticut adopted a sterilization law. The best resources are several surveys conducted by advocates of the bills. A study conducted by a Rhode Island official was particularly rich in information about voting, veto messages, and the positions adopted by key state officials.[1] Of special value is the work of Harry Hamilton Laughlin (who is discussed in Chapter 5), superintendent of the Eugenics Record Office at Cold Spring Harbor, New York, who periodically conducted in-depth surveys of the various states. His book, *Eugenical Sterilization in the United States*, includes an exhaustive legal history of sterilization.[2]

Supporters and Opponents of Sterilization Legislation

Major support for early sterilization laws came from four small but influential segments of society: physicians, especially those working in state institutions; a handful of prominent scientists such as David Starr Jordan, a biologist who was president of Stanford University, and Davenport at Cold Spring Harbor; nonscientific eugenicists (including judges, lawyers, and journalists) who were convinced that eugenics offered a solution to the social problems with which they were so familiar; and wealthy philanthropists, such as Mrs. E. H. Harriman and John D. Rockefeller. I have already discussed the role played by institutionally based physicians and, to some extent, that of the scientific eugenicists. A brief discussion of the other figures in the policy debate is warranted.

While the work of men like Davenport and Goddard provided the scientific basis for a pro-sterilization argument, prominent lawyers, journalists, and business people helped put it before legislators and the public. An example of such an advocate is Warren W. Foster, senior judge of the Court of General Sessions of the County of New York. In November 1909 *Pearson's Magazine,* a widely circulated periodical, published his article titled "Hereditary Criminality and Its Certain Cure." Foster first asserted that sterilization was the best means of stemming the rising tide of criminals. Then the eminent judge assured his readers that a sterilization law would be constitutionally acceptable. A sterilization bill was enacted in New York three years later.[3]

Editorials favoring sterilization were frequently published by popular scientific journals. For example, in June 1911 the editors of *Scientific American* reminded their readers that "the scientific students of mankind, the directors of insane asylums and hospitals, criminologists the world over, have been compiling statistics to show not only the danger of permitting the marriage of criminals, lunatics and the physically unfit, but the effect upon mankind." In their view, "The proper attitude to be taken toward the perpetuation of poor types is . . . You may live, but you must not propagate."[4] *Scientific American*'s editors spoke out in favor of eugenics on at least five occasions during the period 1911-14.

Perhaps the most curious aspect of the eugenics movement was the unusual interest it evoked among America's great industrial families. The support provided by Mrs. Harriman, one of America's wealthiest women, was extraordinary. Besides providing more than fifteen thousand dollars to start the Eugenics Record Office, she guaranteed the salaries of most of the employees. During the early years (1910-12), she gave the ERO about fifteen hundred dollars each month, which covered about four-fifths of its operating costs. Through her lawyer, C. C. Tegethoff, she kept a watchful eye on Cold Spring Harbor. On occasion she even sailed her yacht out to Long Island for a visit. So keen was her interest that Davenport kept her closely informed of the day-to-day operations.[5] During this same period, John D. Rockefeller contributed about four hundred dollars each month, making him the second biggest source of support for the ERO.[6]

Other examples of the enthusiasm with which America's leading families embraced the eugenics movement abound. In 1914 Dr. John Harvey Kellogg, brother of the cereal magnate, organized the First Race Betterment Conference in Battle Creek, Michigan—at that time the largest symposium on eugenics ever held in the United States. Kellogg's interest in eugenics grew, and he eventually started Battle Creek College as a special institution devoted to eugenic education.[7] Samuel Fels, a prominent Philadelphia soap manufacturer, was also a heavy contributor to eugenic causes.

Theodore Roosevelt was another ardent eugenicist. His concern for the ability of the American people to triumph in military conflict led him to embrace positive eugenics. For Roosevelt the essence of national strength depended on a large, healthy population, and he frequently warned the American people about the dangers of "race-suicide." He never tired of advocating the strenuous outdoor life, and he regularly advised his fellow citizens on the importance of having large families. Although he was mainly worried about the deleterious effects on the nation caused by the influx of immigrants, Roosevelt also favored the sterilization of American defectives.[8]

Many other families that were only slightly less prominent also supported eugenics activities. Bleecker Van Wagenen, the chairman of the America Breeders Association's Committee on Sterilization, was a wealthy real estate investor. Madison Grant, a New York lawyer, naturalist, and protector of the city parks, was also a zealous opponent of immigration. His book, *The Passing of the Great Race*, was a manifesto for persons opposed to immigration.[9] The staunchest advocates of sterilization clearly included some immensely powerful people, individuals who could reach the ears of elected officials.

As the call for sterilization laws became more strident, those opposed to such a policy also spoke out. Perhaps the most famous was Franz Boas, a professor of anthropology at Columbia University. In 1907, a year of heightened concern over immigration, Congress created a special Immigration Commission and charged it with determining whether the hordes of newcomers could fit into American society. The commission asked Professor Boas to study the assimilation issue. Reasoning that changes in stature and habitus would be the most easily measured, Boas spent two years measuring immigrants and their American-born children in the streets of New York City. In December 1909 he completed his report entitled *Changes in Bodily Form of Descendants of Immigrants,* which the commission approved and transmitted to Congress. It concluded that Hebrews and Sicilians were easily assimilable, a finding that was anathema to eugenicists.[10]

Alexander Johnson, secretary of the National Conference of Charities and Correction in 1909, was another major critic. He argued that sterilization should not be performed on persons who were so retarded that they would spend their lives in segregated institutions anyway, and that sterilizing criminals would only encourage licentiousness. Instead, Johnson dreamed of establishing, "in every state of the Union, orderly celibate communities segregated from the body politic, set off by themselves on land selected for that purpose, in buildings constructed to some extent by their own hands, where the feeble-minded people, and the epileptic people, and the chronically insane people may be cared for permanently, and a large part of them made entirely self-supporting."[11] Like Johnson, who felt that his opposition to sterilization was a voice "crying in the wilderness," Boas worried that "nature, not nurture, has been raised to the rank of dogma." But even Boas conceded that it was proper "to suppress those defective classes whose deficiencies can be proved by rigid methods to be due to hereditary causes."[12]

Lester Ward, one of the founders of American sociology, effectively debunked the eugenics movement and dismissed its proposals as the fantasies of elitists. But his writings were aimed at academic circles and did not reach a large audience.[13] The editors of the *New York Times* also regularly opposed the more radical eugenics notions. For example, Foster's article in *Pearson's Magazine* provoked an editorial, "Race Homicide," that directly opposed sterilization laws. It gives some picture of the support that the sterilization idea had received:

> When such able and respected men as Judge Warren W. Foster, Judge Charles W. Beckett, and President Eugene Smith of the Prison Association of this State appear to favor a plan that, if adopted by the New York Legislature, as it has already been adopted in Connecticut and Indiana, would condemn before their birth the children of criminals and would prevent their birth, it is time to inquire just how far the State may go in deciding the fate of the future generations. We ask Judge Foster, Judge Beckett and President Smith to reconsider their proposal.[14]

A 1911 report of the Massachusetts Commission to Investigate the Question of the Increase of Criminals, Mental Defectives, Epileptics and Degenerates contains most of the arguments of those opposed to sterilization. The commission doubted the wonderful changes in temperament said to be caused by vasectomy, and it worried that paroling sterilized persons would be a "direct encouragement to sexual vice" leading to an epidemic of venereal disease. It viewed the benefits of vasectomy as unproven and advised the state to adopt a policy of "permanent segregation."[15]

State Sterilization Legislation, 1905-1922

The creation of special commissions to investigate the wisdom of sterilizing defective persons suggests that the sterilization debate was vigorous. Although there is little trace of all the energy that lawmakers devoted to the matter, we do know that between 1905 and 1922, thirty bills permitting the sterilization of institutionalized persons were passed in eighteen states (table 2 lists the most significant ones). The governors of five states (Pennsylvania, Oregon, Vermont, Nebraska, and Idaho) vetoed some of these bills, but laws were eventually enacted during this period in fifteen states. Several states (notably California, which voted favorably on sterilization bills on five occasions between 1909 and 1917) enacted two or more laws on the subject.

Table 2 indicates the legislative vote on these proposals. Although these data give some insight into the public's attitude about sterilization, they are distorted by the fact that we do not know the votes in states that rejected such bills. Nevertheless, it is clear that the states enacting such laws usually did so by a substantial margin. Of the seventeen Senate roll calls listed, the bill passed by a majority of at least two-thirds in all but three. Of the eighteen House roll calls listed, the bill passed by a two-thirds vote in all but four. In the majority of legislatures, the vote was overwhelmingly favorable. With the exception of Vermont, the governors' vetoes probably contradicted popular sentiment. Sterilization advocates had their greatest success in a five-year span from 1909 through 1913. Four of the state laws were enacted in 1913. During this era the sterilization option was also viewed more favorably in the Midwest and Far West than along the Eastern seaboard or in the South or Southwest. Sterilization laws were enacted in three contiguous states in the Northeast, in four contiguous states in the Far West, and in a cluster of eight Midwestern states.[16]

The Indiana and California laws are of special significance. Enacted in 1907, the Indiana statute, which provided a model for other states, firmly

Table 2   State Voting Records on Sterilization Bills, 1905-1921

State	Year	House Vote	Senate Vote	Veto
Pennsylvania	1905	Pass	Pass	Yes
	1921	Pass	36-5	Yes
Indiana	1907	59-22	28-16	
Oregon	1909	50-5	20-10	Yes
	1917	37-18	16-12	
Washington	1909	Pass	Pass	
	1921	68-13	36-1	
California	1909	41-0	21-1	
Connecticut	1909	130-28	Pass	
Iowa	1911	64-13	32-0	
New Jersey	1911	33-6	12-0	
Nevada	1912	34-7	17-1	
New York	1912	78-9	48-0	
North Dakota	1913	73-20	34-4	
Michigan	1913	72-16	21-9	
Kansas	1913	Pass	Pass	
Wisconsin	1913	39-37	24-3	
Vermont	1913	96-82	Pass	Yes
Nebraska	1913	52-33	28-2	Yes
	1915	52-35	21-12	
South Dakota	1918	81-4	34-9	
Idaho	1919	56-1	31-1	Yes

embraced the hereditarian thesis and authorized physicians working at state institutions to sterilize inmates for whom the board of managers agreed that procreation was "inadvisable." Because it greatly influenced later legislation, I quote it completely.

> AN ACT to prevent procreation of confirmed criminals, idiots, imbeciles, and rapists; Providing that superintendents or boards of managers of institutions where such persons are confined shall have the authority and are empowered to appoint a committee of experts, consisting of two physicians, to examine into the mental condition of such inmates.
>
> WHEREAS, heredity plays a most important part in the transmission of crime, idiocy, and imbecility:
>
> THEREFORE, BE IT ENACTED BY THE GENERAL ASSEMBLY OF THE STATE OF INDIANA, that on and after the passage of this act it shall be compulsory for each and every institution in the state, entrusted with the care of confirmed criminals, idiots, rapists and imbeciles, to appoint upon its staff, in addition to the regular institutional physician, two (2) skilled surgeons of recognized ability, whose duty it shall be, in conjunction with the chief physician of the

institution, to examine the mental and physical condition of such inmates as are recommended by the institutional physician and board of experts and the board of managers. If in the judgment of this committee of experts pro-creation is inadvisable, and there is no probability of improvement of the mental and physical condition of the inmate, it shall be lawful for the surgeons to perform such operation for the prevention of procreation as shall be decided safest and most effective. But this operation shall not be performed except in cases that have been pronounced unimproveable. Provided that in no case the consultation fee be more than three dollars to each expert, to be paid out of the funds appropriated for the maintenance of such institution.[17]

California enacted its first sterilization law in February 1909. Like Indiana, it gave institutional physicians broad powers to review inmate records and to sterilize those whom they decided would benefit from the procedure. Special emphasis was placed on sterilizing prisoners. Four years later the statute was replaced by a more expansive law that made two important additions. Patients determined by the "state commission in lunacy" to be suffering from certain mental illnesses could be discharged only upon agreeing to submit to sterilization. The new law also specifically permitted the sterilization of retarded persons ("idiots"), but conditioned surgery upon the written consent of parents or guardians. The consent provision may be one reason why the law was not subjected to constitutional attack. Since more than twenty thousand institutionalized persons were sterilized pursuant to the California law, the key text is presented.

SECTION 1. Before any person who has been lawfully committed to any state hospital for the insane, or who has been an inmate of the Sonoma State Home, and who is afflicted with hereditary insanity or incurable chronic mania or dementia shall be released or discharged therefrom, the State Commission on Lunacy may in its discretion, after a careful investigation of all the circumstances of the case, cause such a person to be asexualized, and such asexualization, whether with or without the consent of the patient, shall be lawful and shall not render said commission, its members or any person participating in the operation liable either civilly or criminally.

SECTION 2. Whenever in the opinion of the resident physician of any state prison it will be beneficial and conducive to the benefit of the physical, mental or moral condition of any recidivist lawfully confined in such state prison to be asexualized, then such physician shall call in consultation the general superintendent of state hospitals and the secretary of the state board of health, and they shall jointly examine into the particulars of the case with the said resident physician, and if in their opinion or the opinion of any two of them, asexualization will be beneficial to such recidivist, they may perform the same; provided, that such operation shall not be performed unless the said recidivist has been committed to a state prison in this or some other state or country at least two times for rape, assault with intent to commit rape, or seduction, or at least three times for any other crime or crimes, and shall have given evidence while an inmate of a state prison in this state that he is a moral or sexual degenerate or pervert; and *provided, further,* that in the case of convicts sentenced to state prison for life, who exhibit continued evidence of moral and sexual depravity, the right to asexualize them, as provided in this section, shall apply whether they shall have been inmates of a state prison in this or any other country or state more than one time or not; provided, further, that nothing in this act shall apply to or refer to any voluntary patient confined or kept in any state hospital of this state.

SECTION 3. Any idiot, if a minor, may be asexualized by or under the direction of the medical superintendent of any state hospital, with the written consent of his or her parent or guardian, and if an adult, then with the written consent of his or her lawfully appointed guardian, and upon the written request of the parent or guardian or any such idiot or fool, the superintendent of any state hospital shall perform such operation or cause the same to be performed without charge therefor.[18]

The term *asexualization* is used here as a synonym for sterilization. California lawmakers did not intend to castrate recidivists and idiots. The word was often misunderstood, and in a few states sterilization proposals may have failed because of opposition to castration.

Although there was great disparity in the level of activity, most states with enabling legislation did implement sterilization programs. Between 1907, when the first law was enacted, and the last day of 1921, there were at least 3,233 sterilizations performed in this nation on institutionalized persons pursuant to state law. A total of 1,853 males and 1,380 women (100 by ovariectomy) were sterilized. The vast majority of these procedures were performed on the insane (2,700) as opposed to the feeble-minded (403) or criminal (130). These figures reflect the fact that in California the insane were far more likely than the retarded to be discharged, and deinstitutionalization was contingent upon sterilization.

As is clear from the number of sterilizations reported by each state during the period 1907-21, even though the leaders of the eugenics movement were situated in the New York area, sterilization was routinely performed only in a few Midwestern states, Oregon, and California. Analysis of statewide patterns of sterilization indicates that programs waxed and waned according to the attitudes of the governors, officials of the relevant state agencies, and superintendents of the particular institutions, and with the judicial resolution of constitutional challenges. For example, during 1907 and 1908 Indiana sterilized 120 (118 men, 2 women) institutional-

Table 3 Sterilizations, 1907-1921

State	Sterilizations	Years Law In Force
California	2,558	1909-1921
Connecticut	27	1909-1921
Indiana[a]	120	1907-1919
Iowa[b]	49	1911-1914, 1915-1921
Kansas	54	1913-1921
Michigan[a]	1	1913-1918
Nebraska	155	1915-1921
Nevada	0	1915-1921
New Jersey[a]	0	1911-1913
New York[a]	42	1912-1918
North Dakota	23	1913-1921
Oregon[c]	127	1913, 1917-1921
South Dakota	0	1917-1921
Washington	1	1909-1912, 1921
Wisconsin	76	1913-1921
Total	3,233	

[a]Law declared unconstitutional during this period.
[b]Law declared unconstitutional in 1913; replaced in 1915.
[c]An Oregon statute enacted in 1913 was repealed by public referendum a few months later. Sterilizations were performed during the period 1917-21, pursuant to a 1917 statute.

ized persons, but in 1909 Governor Thomas Marshall ordered the superintendent of the Jeffersonville Reformatory (the only state institution where the surgery was performed) to stop. During Marshall's tenure, no funds were appropriated to pay for these operations. The Indiana program went unfunded from 1909 until 1919, when it was held to be unconstitutional. Nevertheless, Dr. Sharp continued to sterilize prisoners at Jeffersonville well after 1909.[19]

When sterilization data are analyzed by institution, the influence of the superintendents is readily apparent. In Wisconsin, which permitted eugenic sterilization of "criminal, insane, feeble-minded and epileptic" persons, there were eleven institutions, but (probably for financial reasons) the State Board of Control authorized operations only at the Home for the Feeble-Minded in Chippewa Falls. Dr. A. W. Wilmarth, the superintendent who authorized the sterilization of seventy-six persons between 1913 and 1921, did so because so many "high-grade imbeciles" were sexually active, and to ease the concerns of families when their daughters went home for holiday visits.[20] Concern to protect the feeble-minded girl from pregnancy after seduction or rape by a nonretarded male is a recurring theme in institutional records.

Most New York state officials were reluctant to implement sterilization programs, and in twenty-seven of the thirty institutions covered by its law, no sterilizations took place. But at the State Hospital at Buffalo, where Dr. Arthur W. Hurd believed that childbearing brought on "recurrent attacks of insanity," twelve young schizophrenic women were sterilized. Similarly, at the Gowanda State Hospital, where the superintendent believed that without the burdens of pregnancy some insane women could live successfully in the community, twenty-nine women were sterilized.[21]

Believing that sterilization sometimes allowed insane persons to be placed safely in the community, Dr. F. W. Hatch, general superintendent of the California State Commission on Lunacy, hoped that on occasion vasectomy and salpingectomy might even be curative. Concerned about legal challenges to his eugenics program, Hatch forbade sterilization unless a family member consented in writing (an element *not* required by the statute). As Hatch controlled the selection of superintendents for all state hospitals, it is likely that during his long tenure he hired only advocates of sterilization.[22] During 1915-16, a typical period in the Hatch era, 291 persons (161 men, 130 women) were sterilized, allegedly because each was afflicted with one of the following supposedly Mendelian (genetic) conditions: manic-depressive illness, schizophrenia, epilepsy, imbecility, or drug and alcohol abuse. In 1918 Dr. Charles A. Robinson also reported that by sterilizing a young man at the Preston School of Industry, he had cured the patient of chronic masturbation.[23]

The main goal of the California sterilization program was to prevent the transmission of insanity. This is in marked contrast to other states where the focus was on reducing the incidence of mental retardation. In a single institution, the South California State Hospital (for the insane) in Patton, there were 1,009 persons sterilized in the years prior to 1921. Since this was 40 percent of the national total at that time, Dr. John Reily, the medical superintendent who in a 1918 letter described himself as extremely busy, having "sterilized 43 persons in March," must have been the champion eugenic engineer of his era in the United States.[24] In contrast to the practice at state hospitals, only seven residents of California prisons were sterilized during this period.

The Constitutional Attack on the Statutes

The impressive number of laws enacted between 1909 and 1913 suggests that eugenic sterilization programs enjoyed broad public support and faced little sustained opposition. As I have shown, bills providing for the sterilization of institutionalized persons usually were approved by a substantial majority of the legislatures in both houses. In only three (Wisconsin, Vermont, and Nebraska) of the sixteen legislatures that passed such bills was the vote reasonably close in either of the two houses. These votes were taken in 1913, and the governors of Vermont and Nebraska later vetoed the bills.

The legislative victories did not always translate into active sterilization programs. Except for those in California, and, to some extent, Indiana, Oregon, and Nebraska (where in 1915 a second effort to enact a sterilization law succeeded), relatively few sterilizations were performed prior to World War I. The numerous lawsuits filed against the new statutes substantiate that there was a determined opposition. A successful legal attack on these laws neutralized the legislative victories of those who favored sterilization. Between 1912 and 1921 constitutional challenges were leveled against eight eugenic statutes, and seven were overturned. Analysis of the cases offers some insight into the flaws in the statutes.

The Supreme Court of the State of Washington was the first to rule on the constitutionality of a sterilization statute. The challenge was brought on behalf of a man named Peter Feilen who had been convicted of rape. The trial judge sentenced Feilen to a prison term and, exercising his authority under a new section of the penal code, ordered him to undergo a vasectomy. The statute in question provided that "whenever any person shall be adjudged guilty of carnal abuse of a female person under the age of ten years, or of rape, or shall be adjudged to be an habitual criminal, the court may, in addition to such other punishment or confinement as may be imposed, direct an operation to be performed upon such person for the prevention of procreation." Feilen challenged the power of the state to order him to undergo a vasectomy, arguing that it was a cruel and unusual punishment. In a brief opinion that characterized sterilization purely as a punitive rather than a eugenic measure, the court refused to find that vasectomy was cruel or unusual. The appellate opinion suggests that the court was influenced by Dr. Sharp's testimony that the operation was simple, quick, and painless. Given the court's description of Feilen's crime as "brutal, heinous and revolting," the justices probably had little inclination to spare him. Feilen may be the only convicted rapist ever sterilized under a punitive statute. The Washington law was repealed in 1913, and the sterilization statute that replaced it in 1921 did not apply to convicted criminals.[25]

The only other punitive sterilization statute was enacted in Nevada in 1915. It too provided that persons convicted of child molestation or rape and persons adjudged to be habitual criminals could be subjected to sterilization, but castration was forbidden. In 1918 Pearley C. Mickle, a convicted rapist, challenged a court sterilization order as a violation of the state constitution's prohibition of cruel or unusual punishments. The trial judge, who had invoked the new statute for the first time, had been impressed that Mickle was an epileptic, a diagnosis that he thought predisposed people to commit crimes. Although the appellate court suggested that applying eugenic measures only to institutionalized epileptics violated the Equal Protection Clause of the Fourteenth Amendment, it invalidated the law on other grounds, ruling that vasectomy was an "unusual punishment," prohibited by the Nevada Constitution.[26]

The other six constitutional challenges (New Jersey, Iowa, Michigan, New York, Indiana, and Oregon) were brought against laws that had been intended both to protect the state from the burden of caring for the children born to a defective parent and to enhance the possibility of successfully discharging persons from institutional care. Opponents mounted a two-pronged attack, arguing that the laws, which permitted the sterilization of persons in state institutions, but not similarly affected noninstitutionalized persons, violated the Equal Protection Clause and that they violated the Due Process Clause (no state "shall deprive any person of life, liberty or property without due process of law"). In New Jersey, Michigan, and New York the courts seemed more concerned about inequitable application, while in Iowa, Indiana, and Oregon the judges focused on due process issues. This distinction is important. Those state courts that found the laws in violation of the Equal Protection Clause may not necessarily have opposed involuntary sterilization in principle. Those who overturned the laws on the grounds that they violated the Due Process Clause probably favored a system of safeguards that would have greatly increased the cost of implementing such laws, a position that may have reflected a fundamental antagonism toward such legislation.

The Supreme Court of New Jersey was the first to consider the constitutionality of a eugenic sterilization statute. Entitled "An Act to Authorize and Provide for the Sterilization of Feeble-minded (Including Idiots, Imbeciles and Morons), Epileptics, Rapists, Certain Criminals and Other Defectives," the law was the handiwork of several prominent eugenicists, including David F. Weeks, the aforementioned chief physician of the New Jersey State Village for Epileptics. The law created a Board of Examiners whose duty was to examine the mental and physical condition of appropriate inmates. If the Board of Examiners and the chief physician of an institution unanimously found that procreation was "inadvisable" and that there was no chance that the condition of a particular inmate could improve, it was lawful for the board to order sterilization.

In May 1912 the Board of Examiners and Dr. Weeks approved the sterilization of Alice Smith, an epileptic who had been committed to the State Village in 1902. After a trial court upheld the decision, the lawyer who had been appointed to represent Alice Smith appealed the sterilization order. In reviewing the trial record, the appellate court was impressed that Smith had not had a seizure in five years. It also noted that abdominal surgery would expose the woman to a significant risk of injury or death. After the intermediate-level court overturned the law, another appeal took it to the state supreme court. The justices asked a list of questions. Epilepsy was not the only disease that generated immense social costs. If this law was upheld, could the state sterilize persons with tuberculosis or syphilis? What of nonmedical conditions that society judged undesirable? In a prescient moment, the high court worried that "racial differences, for instance, might afford a basis for such an opinion in the communities where that question is unfortunately a permanent and a paramount issue." By focusing on epileptics who were inmates of state institutions, did not the law ignore the vast majority of similarly affected persons who were at large? As persons in state institutions were segregated by sex and unlikely to procreate, the court reasoned that the law fell on the very group *least* likely to transmit defective germ plasm. It held that the New Jersey law unconstitutionally violated the principle of equal protection before the law.[27]

Shortly after it was enacted in 1913, the constitutionality of Iowa's sterilization law was also challenged. Like others it gave the state board of parole, acting in concert with the managing officer and physician of each public institution, discretionary power to sterilize. That power was to be exercised upon those persons who "would produce children with tendency to disease, deformity, crime, insanity, feeble-mindedness, idiocy, imbecility, epilepsy, or alcoholism, or if the physical or mental condition of any such inmate will probably be materially improved thereby, or if such inmate is an epileptic or syphilitic, or gives evidence, while an inmate of such institution, that he or she is a moral or sexual pervert." The law also made sterilization mandatory for persons convicted of specific sexual offenses and all twice-convicted felons.

The federal judge who heard the case had little doubt that involuntary sterilization was unconstitutional, but he obviously did not understand surgical sterilization. He characterized castration as "physically more severe," but vasectomy as "much the coarser and more vulgar." He asserted that too much had been made of the differences between the two operations, for "the same shame and humiliation and degradation and mental torture" followed both. He struck down the Iowa statute as a cruel and unusual punishment, a violation of the Due Process Clause, and as a bill of attainder (a law punishing a person without a trial).[28]

The New York lawsuit is of special interest because two of the most prominent eugenicists in the United States testified. In 1912 New York adopted an involuntary sterilization law that permitted the Board of Examiners of Feeble-Minded, Criminals, and Other Defectives to review the cases of institutionalized persons and, when appropriate, recommend sterilization. The law provided counsel to the inmate and required that sterilization orders be reviewed in court. In 1917, perhaps in an effort to expand the sterilization program, the Board of Examiners voted to sterilize an inmate at the Rome Custodial Asylum, an institution housing thirteen hundred feeble-minded persons and led by a superintendent who opposed the surgery. To resolve this policy dispute, the board selected a twenty-two-year-old feeble-minded man named Frank Osborn and created a test case. His lawyer promptly appealed the sterilization order.

At the trial the members of the Board of Examiners acknowledged that they had not studied the effects of vasectomy in detail, a fact that troubled the court. The asylum superintendent, Dr. Francis Bernstein, spoke out strongly against the sterilization policy. He denied the eugenic thesis that the proportion of feeble-minded persons in the state was increasing, and he asserted that Frank Osborn was at no increased risk to sire feeble-minded children unless he married a feeble-minded woman. (It was then widely held that most feeble-mindedness was transmitted as an autosomal recessive disorder.) Bernstein also argued that vasectomy was harmful because it encouraged the high-grade feeble-minded to engage in promiscuous sexual relations.

Charles Davenport and Bleeker Van Wagenen also testified. Surprisingly, Davenport did not speak out in favor of sterilization, instead favoring segregation. Given his deep commitment to eugenics programs and his strong support of Laughlin's sterilization studies, it seems likely that Davenport shaped his testimony with an eye on its political implications. Perhaps sensing defeat, he decided to walk a middle ground. Van Wagenen went only a little further, advocating sterilization if patients were capable of consenting. Since he had strongly favored mandatory sterilization of the feeble-minded a few years earlier, Van Wagenen too may have suppressed his views for strategic reasons. The court was especially concerned that the main purpose of the New York statute was to "save expense to future generations." Fearing that the consequences of mass sterilization would be deinstitutionalization of persons who were not able to care for themselves, it struck down the law as a violation of the Equal Protection Clause.[29]

In 1919, the Supreme Court of Indiana overturned the nation's original eugenic sterilization law. Although Dr. Sharp had perfected the vasectomy on the men of the Jeffersonville Reformatory, since 1909 a series of unsympathetic governors had refused to fund his program. When a test case was brought, the court dismissed the arguments of sterilization advocates without discussion, holding that the law had failed to satisfy minimal standards of due process.[30]

During the years 1918-21, when most of the judicial opinions were handed down, the sterilization laws faded almost as quickly as they had appeared. While there may have been many reasons why the courts were less sympathetic to the notion of sterilization than legislators had been, one was certainly that sterilization orders (like commitment orders) triggered the judiciary's historic role as protector of the weak. The judges demanded clear proof that the feeble-minded or other dependent individual would be helped by the operation. Another reason was that in the few years that elapsed between enactment and invalidation of these laws, scientific challenges to Davenport's simplistic vision of human inheritance began to appear. For example, in 1913 Dr. Edith Spaulding and Dr. William Healy published their study of a thousand cases of young recidivists, a study undertaken to determine to what extent inheritance was really a factor in criminal behavior. At the annual meeting of the American Academy of Medicine in Minneapolis, they argued, "we can find no proof of the existence of hereditary criminalistic traits." They dismissed "the idea of base criminalistic traits, especially in their hereditary aspects, as an unsubstantiated metaphysical hypothesis."[31] Spaulding and Healy were among the first scientists to attack the lurid conclusions about the Jukes, the Kallikaks, and other "degenerate" families. But despite the increasing cracks in its scientific foundation, the triumphant years for eugenic sterilization lay ahead.

5 · Harry H. Laughlin: Champion of Sterilization

No mistakes need be made; for at first only the very lowest would be selected for sterilization, and their selection would be based on the study of their personal and family histories and the individual so selected must first be proved to be the carrier of hereditary traits of a low and menacing order.

—Harry Hamilton Laughlin, 1914

Our studies show also that the compulsory feature is now soundly established in long practice. They show also that the subject for sterilization does not necessarily have to be an inmate of an institution, but may be selected with equal legality from the population at large. It remains to be seen whether the states can extend sterilization to apparently normal individuals who have come from exceedingly inferior stocks, judged by the constitutional qualities of their close kin.

—Harry Hamilton Laughlin, 1932

The history of efforts to secure the involuntary sterilization of defective persons is the history of actions taken by a small but dedicated group of persons who were convinced that the future of the United States depended on protecting the "race." At the center of this group stood Harry Hamilton Laughlin, a schoolteacher from the Midwest, who moved to Cold Spring Harbor in 1910 and became a zealous propagandist for eugenics. Between 1910 and 1939 he worked indefatigably on every issue in the eugenics movement, but his major efforts were rationalizing the strict quotas on the immigration of "weaker" racial stocks and encouraging the sterilization of the unfit.

Harry Hamilton Laughlin was born in Oskaloosa, Iowa, in 1880, but he regarded Kirksville, Missouri, to which his family moved in 1891, as his home. He was the only one of five brothers who did not study osteopathy, choosing instead to qualify as a teacher. After graduating from North Missouri State Normal School in 1900, Laughlin continued his studies at Iowa State College, but received no degree. Between 1900 and 1905 he served as a high school principal and taught biology. From 1905 to 1907 he was the superintendent of schools in Kirksville, leaving that post to teach courses in agriculture at the college from which he had graduated.[1]

The early years of the twentieth century were exciting ones for the agricultural sciences. The rediscovery of Mendel's work promised advances in the breeding of domestic crops and animals. In February 1907, Laughlin, who was conducting breeding experiments with some uncommon varieties of poultry, wrote to Charles Benedict Davenport, director of the new Station for Experimental Evolution at Cold Spring Harbor, for advice on how to classify his animals.[2] This initiated a correspondence that led Laughlin to New York that summer to take a course in genetics, an experience that he later described as "the most profitable six weeks that I have ever spent." Davenport must have liked Laughlin, because he invited him to return the following year, an invitation that Laughlin was unable to accept.[3]

During the ensuing years Laughlin and Davenport communicated regularly. The young instructor certainly scored a coup when he persuaded the well-known scientist to visit the college at Kirksville while traveling to the annual meeting of the American Breeder's Association (ABA) in Columbia, Missouri.[4] Davenport discussed his growing interest in human heredity with Laughlin, whom he easily recruited to work with him. By 1909 Laughlin was busily collecting family data for the "Mendelian blanks" (family pedigree charts) that Davenport sent him.

Laughlin and his wife, Pansy Bowen, a schoolteacher who traced her ancestry to a signer of the Declaration of Independence, returned to Cold Spring Harbor in the summer of 1910. Under Davenport's direction, Laughlin became interested in a project to train "field workers" to gather extensive family histories. It was hoped that this would permit scientists to parse the heritability of "positive" and "negative" human characteristics. Soon after he convinced Mary Harriman to underwrite the creation of a Eugenics Record Office (ERO), Davenport invited Laughlin to become superintendent and assume responsibility for analyzing the family data being collected by the field workers. Laughlin promptly accepted, and in October he and Pansy moved to Cold Spring Harbor. From the first he demonstrated a commitment that never flagged. Davenport's satisfaction is evident in a letter to Mrs. Harriman: "I was surprised to see how receptive he was of the idea. He said there would be no financial advantage but that, above all, he desired to go into this work. He made no condition, even as to the length of his appointment. I am more than ever satisfied that he is the man for us."[5]

During the next four years, Laughlin threw himself into the task of developing the ERO. The most immediate need was to recruit, train, and deploy an army of field workers. The bulk of the training was accomplished through a special summer program. Placement was not difficult; every state institution was eager to host or hire an ERO-trained field worker. By 1911 a small but growing group of dedicated young persons (mostly women) was collecting information about the ancestry of the insane, the feeble-minded, epileptics, and paupers who inhabited those institutions, and sending the data to the ERO. During the next few years the drizzle of information became a torrent.

Laughlin worked tirelessly to analyze and store the data. He developed a method for abstracting the data from large family charts to file cards. These were stored in fireproof cabinets and triple-indexed for easy access. By 1939, when the ERO met its demise, there were hundreds of thousands of entries, perhaps the most extensive genealogical collection ever compiled in the United States save for that of the Mormon church. Today the original cabinets stuffed with neatly filed cards slumber peacefully in the basement of the Dight Institute at the University of Minnesota.

It is difficult to pinpoint precisely when Laughlin become interested in the sterilization of defective persons. Certainly, eugenics was topical during his high school and college years. The fact that he had a mild seizure disorder may explain both his interest in eugenics and his childless marriage. He was unquestionably exposed to arguments favoring sterilization at the meeting of the American Breeder's Association that he attended with Davenport in January 1909. Started in 1903 by W. M. Hays, a professor of plant breeding at the University of Minnesota and a former United States assistant secretary of agriculture, the ABA, an organization of pragmatic farmers and university-based theoreticians, flourished for a time. By 1906 the group had spawned forty-three committees, including one on eugenics chaired by David Starr Jordan, president of Stanford University.[6]

Under the influence of Jordan (who believed that racial degeneration threatened the nation), the committee's goal was stated with some urgency. It hoped to "emphasize the value of superior blood and the menace to society of inferior blood." In 1910, the year in which Davenport was its secretary, the ABA Committee on Eugenics issued a report advocating surgical sterilization of persons identified as potential parents of defective children.[7]

The ABA had become so interested in the problem of racial degeneration that in 1912 it created the Committee to Study and to Report on the

Best Practical Means of Cutting off the Defective Germ Plasm in the American Population. The five-man committee was chaired by Bleeker Van Wagenen, the prominent New York attorney. Harry Laughlin, the only other nonphysician, was named as its secretary. The committee consulted with a blue-ribbon panel of experts that included Dr. Lewellys F. Barker, physician at the Johns Hopkins School of Medicine, Henry H. Goddard, the psychometrician at the Vineland Training School in New Jersey, geneticist Raymond Pearl, and Louis Marshall, a prominent New York lawyer who led the American Jewish Congress. It also undertook a survey of physicians to determine the long-term effects of sterilization. This survey, the first of its kind, was conducted by Laughlin.[8]

At the 1913 meeting of the ABA, Van Wagenen delivered the committee's report. The document, which was among Laughlin's earliest writings on the subject, read in part:

> In recent years society has become aroused to the fact that the number of individuals within its defective classes has rapidly increased both absolutely and in proportion to the entire population; that eleemosynary expenditure is growing yearly; that some normal strains are becoming contaminated with anti-social and defective traits; and that the shame, the moral retardation, and the economic burden of the presence of such individuals are more keenly felt than ever before. Within the last three years especially there has been a marked development of public interest in this matter. The word "Eugenics" has for the first time become known to thousands of intelligent people who now seek to understand its full significance and application. Biologists tell us that whether of wholly defective inheritance or because of an insurmountable tendency toward defect, which is innate, members of the following classes must generally be considered as socially unfit and their supply should if possible be eliminated from the human stock if we would maintain or raise the level of quality essential to the progress of the nation and our race:
>
> 1. The Feeble Minded: using the term generally.
> 2. The Pauper class: pauper families through successive generations.
> 3. The Criminaloids: persons born with marked criminal tendencies.
> 4. Epileptics.
> 5. The Insane: (excepting certain forms of acute insanity showing no hereditary taint).
> 6. The Constitutionally Weak, or asthenic class.
> 7. Those predisposed to specific diseases or the diathetic class.
> 8. The Congenitally Deformed.
> 9. Those having defective sense organs, such as the deaf-mutes, the deaf and the blind, or the Kakaisthetic class.
>
> With the statistics at present available it is impossible to give an accurate

statement of the numbers within each of these classes in the United States. From studies of such figures of the 11th, 12th and 13th U.S. special Censuses as a basis, it seems safe to conclude that nearly 1% of the total population is under custodial care and control in institutions all the time. This is a shifting and constantly changing population so that many more than that number in the aggregate are inmates of institutions in the course of any one year. Outside of institutions it seems conservative to estimate from $3\frac{1}{2}$% to 4% equally defective persons not under custodial care, while upon the borderline, just above this class there are probably several millions (perhaps four to five millions) or say 5% more who are barely able to maintain themselves or who just succeed in abstaining from acts which would bring them into the custody of the State. These are so interwoven in kinship with those still more defective that they are wholly unfitted to become the parents of useful and valuable citizens. They carry germ plasm more or less charged with defects and unless their matings are with better strains deterioration is sure to follow in their family lines. Thus, we conclude that approximately 10% of our population, primarily through inherent defect and weakness, are an economic and moral burden on the 90% and a constant source of danger to the national and racial life. It is impossible to measure the industrial and social handicap caused by these individuals. But just as the leaders of successful human endeavor exert an influence altogether incommensurate with their number, so this class, doubtless, constitute a drag on society of similar magnitude.[9]

Of the ten possible solutions to the problem of defective germ plasm that the committee considered (ranging from segregation to euthanasia), it strongly favored sterilization as the least objectionable and most cost-effective method. This was because of the findings of its sterilization survey, which included interviews with Dr. Sharp's patients in Indiana. Although the Van Wagenen Report was the most thorough argument in favor of sterilization produced in the United States, it probably had little impact on social policy. As we have seen, by 1913 the first wave of sterilization laws had already peaked. Professor Hays died that year, leaving a vacuum in the leadership of the American Breeder's Association. During the war years, the group was reorganized as the American Genetics Association and started a new periodical, the *Journal of Heredity*, which was aimed at the general reader.

For Laughlin, work on the Van Wagenen Committee was immensely important. It stimulated him to amass reams of data about sterilization practices and policies in each of the states, material that he faithfully updated and published in exhaustive detail over the next fifteen years. The first products were two monographs written by him and published by the ERO in 1914. One was a meticulous discussion, *The Legal, Legislative, and*

Administrative Aspects of Sterilization.[10] His remarkably thorough analysis of legislative activity, which included current statutes, proposed bills, and the veto messages of several governors, was merely a beginning. He also conducted a detailed census of sterilization practices within the states, the first of several that he would undertake over the next two decades.

Laughlin gave much thought to the appropriate reach of sterilization laws. The Van Wagenen Committee had conservatively estimated that four-fifths of mental defectives were not housed in institutions. Thus, a narrowly drawn law would fail to encompass the vast majority of the persons who (in its view) should be eugenically sterilized. Laughlin drafted a "model" sterilization law that he hoped would be enacted in every state. Designed to be broad in scope, adequately funded, and above constitutional attack, it proposed a Eugenics Commission, which would systematically review the record of every institutionalized person in the state and decide who had "the potential to produce offspring who, because of the inheritance of inferior or antisocial traits, would probably become a social menace, or a ward of the state." Such persons would be recommended for sterilization, but would have the right to judicial review.

The contacts that Laughlin made while working on the ABA committee helped him emerge as a key figure in the American eugenics movement. An early sign of his growing reputation came when he was invited to address the First National Conference on Race Betterment held at Battle Creek, Michigan, in January 1914. Dr. J. H. Kellogg had started the Battle Creek Sanitarium on the principle that by adopting a carefully regulated life style, individuals might lead healthier lives. By 1914 he had become interested in positive eugenics (programs to breed healthier humans), an interest that led him to organize the conference. Lasting for five days and attended by 406 official delegates and thousands of curious visitors, the conference was the largest of its kind ever held in the United States. Besides eugenics and immigration, the topics included statistical studies of health, individual hygiene, alcohol and tobacco, child life, sex questions, school and industrial hygiene, and city, state, and national hygiene.

Laughlin's lecture, "Calculations on the Working Out of a Proposed Program of Sterilization," asserted that 10 percent of the population was defective. He argued that the threat of the socially inadequate was so severe that neither moral nor economic issues should preclude intervention. He marshaled mountains of statistics to show that their number would increase at a rate that would inevitably destroy the society. This could only be averted if such individuals were institutionalized and if sterilization was made a prerequisite for discharge, thus neutralizing their allegedly high fertility.[11]

The war years (1914-18), a quiet period for American eugenics, constituted a period of consolidation in Laughlin's career. Working in the shadow of several first-rate biologists that Davenport had attracted to the Station for Experimental Evolution may have made him anxious about his scientific credentials. In 1914 Laughlin was accepted for doctoral work in biology at Princeton. Although he only spent one academic year in residence and continued to work at the ERO in 1915 and 1916, Laughlin earned a doctorate in 1917. His dissertation, "On Mitosis in the Root Tip of the Common Onion," was written under the direction of Edward Grant Conklin, a cytologist of national stature.[12] The Princeton degree gave Laughlin a measure of acceptability as a geneticist, but his doctoral project was the only rigorous experimental study that he ever published.[13] Over the next three decades he pursued a quixotic search for methods of breeding a superior racehorse, but papers based on this work were largely speculative. Laughlin thought of himself as a scientist and never argued when journalists referred to him as a geneticist. By carefully cultivating this image he was able to claim no small authority with the press and public, a situation that helped him to press home his views.

Laughlin's Emergence as a Eugenics Expert

As part of his work for the Van Wagenen Committee, Laughlin surveyed most of the institutions for the feeble-minded in the United States. This may have been what prompted officials of the U.S. Census Bureau to engage him to study the residents of the nation's custodial institutions (such as almshouses and schools for the feeble-minded). Commissioned late in 1914, the work was, despite Laughlin's studies at Princeton, nearly complete by March 1916. On March 11, he wrote Davenport that the Bureau was planning to print five thousand copies of the "Statistical Directory of State Institutions for the Socially Inadequate." He also confided that the director did not like the title and had sought unsuccessfully to use a more neutral term to describe the nation's underprivileged.[14]

Publication of the survey of 634 state institutions was delayed for four years. It finally appeared under a similar title: *A Statistical Directory of State Institutions for the Care of Defective, Dependent, and Delinquent Classes.* Nevertheless, the survey was an important event in Laughlin's career. The data that he gathered on the ethnicity of the nation's institutionalized persons convinced him that recent immigrants were hindering rather than helping American society. He moved quickly to disseminate his findings, which confirmed the worst fears of that fraction of the nation opposed to open-door immigration.[15]

From 1917 to 1919 Laughlin devoted most of his energy to writing an opus on eugenic sterilization. By 1919 the work had progressed to the point that Davenport mentioned it in his annual report to the Carnegie Institute, the organization that provided core funding for the ERO.[16] But the manuscript had reached such vast proportions (thirteen hundred pages) and held so little promise of selling well that the Carnegie Institute (which focused on basic science) showed no interest in paying for its publication. Knowing that John D. Rockefeller had underwritten some of the ERO's operational costs, Laughlin next asked Katherine B. Davis, director of the Bureau of Social Hygiene, an organization supported by the Rockefeller Foundation, for help. Although she agreed that the statistical material that he had compiled was valuable, she was troubled by his "direct propaganda favoring sterilization legislation." In a letter written to Raymond D. Fosdick, president of the Rockefeller Foundation, on February 2, 1921, Miss Davis urged that he not provide the seven thousand dollars needed to complete the project.[17]

Despite these setbacks, Laughlin continued to expand the scope of the project, conducting yet another survey, this time of 160 institutions with sterilization programs. A few months later he finally secured the needed financial support. The Chicago Psychopathic Laboratory, a pet project of Judge Harry Olson, chief of the city's criminal court system and a devout believer in hereditary criminality, agreed to publish the book. When the extraordinarily detailed study, *Eugenical Sterilization in the United States,* appeared in 1922, it easily qualified Laughlin as the nation's foremost expert.[18]

During the years that Laughlin was writing his sterilization study, he was also working to limit the influx of immigrants. On April 16 and 17, 1920, he testified before the House Committee on Immigration and Naturalization on the eugenic consequences of immigration. His remarks, based on the survey that he had conducted for the Census Bureau, were music to the ears of a committee that was dominated by opponents of immigration. Laughlin's findings strongly disputed earlier congressional studies that tended to minimize the threat posed by large-scale immigration from southeastern Europe and Russia.

With the onset of World War I, immigration dropped drastically, but in the postwar years the pace rose dramatically and calls for restricting the influx were strident. Strongly restrictionist himself, Laughlin was delighted to testify as the House committee's only scientific witness. His comments, published by the Government Printing Office as a pamphlet entitled *Biological Aspects of Immigration,* were a dire warning that the nation's hospitals and eleemosynary institutions would soon be overwhelmed by immigrants who were unable to care for themselves.[19] Within the year Albert Johnson, chairman of the committee, appointed him "Expert Eugenical Agent." His assignment was to study "alien inmates and inmates of recent foreign extraction in the several state institutions for the socially inadequate." He planned to analyze the relative incidence of defects among foreign-born inmates and compare them to that in the native stock.[20]

His plan was simple. Starting with census data on the proportion of the American population represented by each national group (Italian, Swedish, etc.), Laughlin calculated the number of each group that he expected to find in the institutional population. He then studied ninety-three insane asylums, numerous prisons, and a variety of special facilities (such as tuberculosis sanitariums), gathering and sifting masses of data and compiling an impressive array of charts and graphs. If a greater than expected number of foreign-born persons appeared in his survey of 84,106 inmates, then that national group was contributing a disproportionate share of socially inadequate citizens. Therefore, immigration from that country threatened the racial strength of the American people.

The survey, published as *Analysis of America's Modern Melting Pot*, confirmed the prejudices of the eugenics movement. Laughlin found only 91.89 percent of the expected number of native whites in institutions, but 125.79 percent of the expected number of foreign stock, and 143.24 percent of the expected number of persons of Southern and Eastern European extraction. Laughlin concluded that "making all logical allowances for environmental conditions, which may be unfavorable to the immigrant, the recent immigrants (largely from Southern and Eastern Europe), as a whole, present a higher percentage of inborn social inadequate qualities than do the older stocks."[21]

Completed in the autumn of 1922 and printed as part of the Hearings before the House Committee on Immigration and Naturalization of the 67th Congress, the report was the ammunition that Albert Johnson, now deeply involved in a struggle to secure legislation that would significantly reduce immigration from Eastern Europe, needed to rationalize his views. Since the committee had commissioned no other studies and had limited the testimony before it, Johnson was able to build a staunchly pro-restrictionist record. As Bruno Lasker, editor of *The Survey* put it, "We feel that Dr. Laughlin's arguments for further restriction are difficult to combat if they are true, and that his facts will in the future be thrown at us every time we plead for liberal treatment of the immigration question."[22]

By 1923 Laughlin stood as the leading scientific expert on the biology of immigration. No other authorities seriously or consistently challenged him. So dominant was his position that Dr. Raymond Pearl, a leading geneticist who had repudiated his earlier belief in eugenics, feared "that the opinions of Congressmen generally regarding this group [Laughlin and his colleagues] is that it is the only one which has any scientific knowledge about immigration."[23]

Because it appeared after the Immigration Act of 1921, itself a restrictive measure, had become law, the major impact of Laughlin's report was on the next major legislation. The 1921 law created a quota system keyed to the national origins of the population residing in America in 1910 (the most recent year for which census data were available). It limited the annual immigration of people from each European country to 3 percent of the total number of Americans that had claimed that country as their place of origin in 1910. But this law had been passed as a temporary measure to give Congress time to decide upon a national immigration policy. Further, it was a compromise between a nativist House of Representatives and a more cautious Senate. The Senate needed persuasion.

Laughlin provided the House committee, which was trying to capitalize on a strongly nativist sentiment in the land and in the White House (President Coolidge had bluntly advocated restrictionist measures prior to taking office), with the data that it needed to justify a key change: to switch the reference year from 1910, a time by which many "socially inadequate" types had already emigrated from Italy and Poland, to 1890, when the majority of new immigrants hailed from northwestern Europe, the homeland of the favored Nordic and Teutonic "races." One historian has even argued that Laughlin's report played a critical role in the enactment of the Immigration Act of 1924.[24] Johnson and other committee members were careful not to rant about declining racial vigor. They merely asserted that Laughlin's analysis of institutions indicated which peoples were difficult to assimilate. Would it not be foolish to open our doors to people who were unlikely to adapt to new ways? Besides, the 1890 census reflected the national origins of most Americans. Would it not be unfair to bias immigration policy in favor of the latest wave? Under the cloak of justice, the base year for the 1924 act was shifted from 1910 to 1890, and the annual allowable immigration from Italy, Poland, and Greece was cut by 80 percent. Both the House and the Senate voted overwhelmingly in favor of the bill, which President Coolidge signed. In Laughlin's view, the law undoubtedly did more to prevent the dilution of American racial strength by inferior types than did all the sterilization laws together. It was his greatest triumph.

Fame and Controversy

Although his stature within the eugenics community grew steadily during his first decade (1910-20) at the ERO, Laughlin catapulted to new heights in 1922. That year the Psychopathic Laboratory of the Chicago Municipal Court published his book, *Eugenical Sterilization in the United States,* which included the model law that Laughlin was so sure would survive constitutional scrutiny. In the autumn of 1922 he also completed *Analysis of America's Modern Melting Pot,* which, as we have seen, so greatly influenced Congress. At forty-two, after twelve years in Davenport's shadow, Laughlin was himself a leading eugenicist.

In February 1923 he was elected to the Galton Society, an exclusive club dedicated to the "study of the origin and evolution of man," which met at the American Museum of Natural History. Organized in 1918, the Galton Society represented the inner circle of American eugenics. Davenport, Madison Grant, and Edwin G. Conklin (under whom Laughlin had earned his Princeton degree) were among its charter members. Laughlin was surely ecstatic at achieving some measure of social and intellectual parity with these men. Any one of several accomplishments may have earned him entry to this inner sanctum of eugenically minded intellectuals. Besides having written his impressive work on sterilization and his service to Congress, Laughlin had worked zealously to ensure the success of the Second International Congress of Eugenics, held at the American Museum of Natural History in September of 1921. This commitment may have impressed Henry Fairfield Osborne, president of the congress, who was the director of the museum and an organizer of the Galton Society.

During the next few years Laughlin's star continued to rise. In 1923, with the aid of the Committee on Immigration and Naturalization of the House of Representatives, he secured an appointment from the Department of Labor as Special Immigration Agent to Europe.[25] He then toured Europe for six months to gather more data on the threat posed by immigration. This led to his third congressional report, *Europe as an Emigrant Exporting Continent and the United States as an Immigrant Receiving Nation,* a strongly pro-restrictionist document, but one that probably appeared too late to directly influence the Immigration Restriction Act of 1924.[26]

During the twenties Laughlin conducted annual surveys to monitor implementation of state sterilization laws. In 1926 the newly formed American Eugenics Society, the inner circle of which was dominated by several Yale professors, published Laughlin's 755-page update of his 1922 study. For eugenicists the news was good. A period of quiescence during and after

World War I was giving way to an upsurge both in legislative activity and in the number of eugenic sterilizations. By 1926, twenty-three states had enacted sterilization laws and seventeen had active programs, pursuant to which 6,244 persons had been sterilized.[27]

Besides his duties as superintendent of the ERO, Laughlin had many other commitments. He almost single-handedly edited and wrote much of the copy for *Eugenical News,* a monthly magazine aimed at the general public. In 1920, he wrote twelve columns for the magazine; in 1926, he wrote about fifty; and during the period 1929-31 he wrote well over one hundred columns each year. He also traveled widely to spread the gospel of eugenic sterilization. For example, on May 1, 1926, he lectured to the Kentucky Academy of Medicine, and on June 4 he delivered a paper, "Eugenical Sterilization of the Feeble-Minded," to a meeting of the American Association for the Study of the Feeble-Minded in Toronto.[28]

Laughlin was constantly trying to raise money to support the sterilization movement. During the early 1920s Walter J. Salmon, a wealthy New Yorker, initiated a project with Laughlin to breed the ultimate thoroughbred horse. Laughlin tried repeatedly and unsuccessfully to persuade him to sponsor the proposed Salmon Institution for Eugenical Research, which would study the beneficial effects of sterilization. Laughlin also solicited money from Charles M. Goethe, a wealthy Californian deeply concerned about Mexican immigration, but Goethe gave most of his support to eugenics projects on the West Coast. In 1927, after Harvard University rejected a sixty-thousand-dollar bequest to support instruction in eugenics, Laughlin tracked the court battle over the will, and when the money was awarded to Jefferson Medical College, he again (unsuccessfully) sought a piece of the pie.[29]

Given that other activities brought him more public acclaim, it is ironic that the most important deed that Laughlin performed to further eugenic sterilization was probably to write a letter to a Virginia official in October 1924. In March of that year, Virginia had joined a growing number of states that were enacting laws aimed at sterilizing "potential parents of socially inadequate offspring," the term in Laughlin's model statute. A few months later Carrie Buck, said to be the feeble-minded mother of a feeble-minded child, was committed to a Virginia institution by her adoptive mother. Dr. A. S. Priddy, superintendent of the Lynchburg Colony, a large residential facility, chose her as the test case by which to determine the constitutionality of the new law.[30]

Priddy and Aubrey Strode, the attorney who had guided the Virginia bill into law, first obtained a sterilization order from the board of directors of the Lynchburg Colony and then convinced a friend of Strode's, I. P.

Whitehead, to represent Carrie Buck in the court test. Working carefully to build an airtight record, Priddy wrote to Laughlin to ask him to act as an expert in evaluating Carrie Buck's fitness for sterilization. Laughlin requested a detailed family and personal history, only some of which Priddy was able to supply. Although he was not trained as a physician or as a psychologist and had never met Carrie Buck, Laughlin used Priddy's sketchy material to answer a long set of interrogatories, documents that figured prominently in the judge's decision to uphold the sterilization order. Laughlin opined that Carrie Buck had a mental age of nine, was sexually immoral, and was a typical "low-grade moron." He considered the possibility that she was feeble-minded due to environmental rather than hereditary causes to be "exceptionally remote."[31]

Laughlin's conclusion that Carrie Buck was the "potential parent of socially inadequate offspring," along with testimony by Dr. A.H. Estabrook, a fellow Carnegie Institute scientist (and author of *The Jukes in 1915*), and Dr. Joseph de Jarnette, superintendent of another Virginia institution, who testified (erroneously) that feeble-mindedness was a Mendelian disorder, built a convincing record. Carrie Buck's attorney called no medical experts, focusing his attack on issues of due process. The new law was upheld by the Virginia Supreme Court and the Supreme Court of the United States.[32] Although the case did not receive much publicity, it heralded a new era. Until the Supreme Court decision, state sterilization programs had been operating on a relatively modest scale. But after *Buck v. Bell* (discussed more fully in Chapter 7), the pace picked up and did not slacken until World War II.

During the late 1920s and early 1930s, Laughlin's work became international in scope. In 1928 he went to Havana as an adviser to Cuba at the Second International Conference on Emigration and Immigration. In 1930 he was secretary of the Third International Congress of Eugenics, which met in London. He continued to act as sole "eugenics expert" for the House Committee on Immigration and Naturalization, and he generated a steady stream of reports that reinforced the restrictionist cause.[33]

Although Laughlin's stature with the nation's scientific community was sufficient to secure an invitation to join the National Research Council Committee on Human Heredity in 1929, even then he was under attack for drawing overly broad and poorly supported conclusions from his research. Not a few scientists and policy makers must have worried that his work was overtly prejudiced. As early as 1914, a student at the ERO training program for field workers complained to Mrs. Harriman that Laughlin had discriminated against him because he was Jewish.[34] Shortly after the U.S.

Congress published Laughlin's *Analysis of America's Melting Pot,* Dr. John C. Merriam, president of the Carnegie Institute, began to complain to Davenport that Laughlin's work was laden with prejudice.[35] In October of that year, Merriam (who controlled ERO funding) again was angered by criticisms leveled in *Nature* at Laughlin's work on sterilization. In 1929 he rebuked Laughlin for using ERO stationery to lobby Congress.[36] Although Dr. Merriam's dissatisfaction with Laughlin grew as the years passed, he apparently had a long fuse. It was not until after Davenport's retirement that Laughlin's position at the ERO became precarious.

During the early 1930s Laughlin, convinced that eugenicists had won the sterilization battle (needing only to increase the rate at which operations were performed), returned to the immigration problem. In 1933 and 1934 there was considerable debate over whether the Immigration Act of 1924 should be amended to allow more Jews to leave Germany for asylum in the United States. The Executive Board of the Chamber of Commerce of the State of New York, which convened a special committee to review the matter, asked Laughlin to study the question. Laughlin's report, which was adopted by the committee and mailed to all members of the New York State Chamber of Commerce, concluded that there should be "no exceptional admission for Jews who are refugees from persecution in Germany." As he put it: "The Jews are no exception to races which are widely variable in family-stock quality within their own race. There are superior Jews and there are inferior Jews . . . . High grade Jews are welcome and low-grade Jews must be excluded." Laughlin was more concerned by the threat posed to the United States by the immigration of inferior persons than the risks that Jews faced in Nazi Germany. He feared that if the United States continued to be the world's asylum and poorhouse, it would soon wreck its economic life and its future inheritance.[37] In August of 1934, Laughlin completed yet another survey of foreign-born inmates of American institutions, and again offered his findings as evidence to support a tight immigration policy. The *Saturday Evening Post* applauded his views.[38]

Although Laughlin remained popular with some members of the press and continued to receive invitations to lead various study groups, Doctor Merriam steadily lost patience with his work. In 1935 he sought the opinion of L. C. Dunn, a highly regarded geneticist, about eugenics in general and Laughlin in particular. Dunn replied that many geneticists were quite critical of eugenicists because their research "was not always activated by purely disinterested scientific motives."[39] But it was not until 1938 that Merriam, about to retire from the Carnegie Institute, decided to get rid of Laughlin. Rejecting the perfunctory annual letter from a physician attesting to Laughlin's good health, Merriam demanded a second opinion. He then cut Laughlin's funding by 80 percent and guaranteed his salary for only the first quarter of 1939.[40] Laughlin had no choice but to resign.

The Carnegie Institute, repudiating its past interest in eugenics, promptly closed the Eugenics Record Office. The hundreds of thousands of family file cards were shipped to the University of Minnesota, and Laughlin's massive personal papers were sent in a boxcar to his home in Kirksville, Missouri.[41] After his death in 1942, these papers became the property of Northeast Missouri State University, where they still reside.

6 · The Resurgence of Eugenics

Shall America head for race suicide or for race improvement?
—W. A. Plecker, Virginia State Registrar of Vital Statistics, 1925

"Law Defining 'Black Blood' in La. Upheld"
—(New Orleans) Times-Picayune/The States, May 19, 1983

As we have seen, in the first two decades of this century a remarkable number of sterilization laws were enacted, and about thirty-two hundred institutionalized persons were subjected to eugenic sterilization. The bulk of this activity took place from 1909 to 1913, and legislative voting records suggest that the laws had wide support. However, eugenic sterilization programs were actually implemented only in those states in which key persons, such as superintendents of state hospitals, were supportive. Except in California and several Midwestern states, relatively few residents of institutions were sterilized. During World War I, many of the laws were struck down by the courts, and for a time (1918-22), no new sterilization statutes were enacted.

Despite the demise of most of the laws, the number of institutionalized persons who were sterilized each year in the United States continued to rise. This was largely due to the California program. From January 1, 1918, until December 31, 1920, there were 1,150 sterilizations performed upon persons in six California state hospitals for the insane, roughly one for every six persons admitted. About three hundred retarded persons were also sterilized at the Sonoma State Home, an institution with a capacity of twenty-two hundred residents. During those three years, approximately 80 percent of all eugenic sterilizations carried out in the United States were performed in seven institutions in one state.[1]

Despite the quiescence of sterilization programs virtually everywhere except California, the sterilization movement soon made a remarkable comeback. A small number of eugenicists capitalized effectively on the national concern over the dramatic postwar influx of immigrants from

Southern and Eastern Europe and growing uneasiness about the northern migration of American blacks. The resurgence of sterilization programs was closely tied to the popular demand to limit immigration. The eugenicists' argument that hordes of immigrants would weaken the American gene pool provided part of the intellectual rationale for the restrictive Immigration Act of 1924. It is no accident that a second wave of state sterilization laws, targeted at a different threat to the "race," were enacted at the same time.

The issues discussed at the Second International Congress of Eugenics, which met at the American Museum of Natural History in New York City in September 1921, reflect this dual concern. Authorities in genetics, medicine, and eugenics presented 108 papers. Fifty-three reported on laboratory genetics or pedigree studies that documented the inheritance of human traits;[2] 55 addressed the biological and social consequences of marriages between persons of different ethnic backgrounds.[3] As the papers, including those such as "Some Notes on the Negro Problem," "The Problem of Negro-White Intermixture," and "Inter-marriage with the Slave Race" suggest, there was special concern about miscegenation. Nor was that concern limited to eugenic circles. During the first quarter of this century, many states enacted laws that were intended to tighten already existing limits on interracial marriage.

The roots of antimiscegenation law are deeply set in the soil of American history. As early as 1630, only a few years after Negroes were brought to Virginia, the governor's council declared that Hugh Davis, a white man, was to be whipped publicly for "abusing himself to the dishonor of God and shame of Christians by defiling his body in lying with a Negro." In 1662, the state's general antifornication statute was amended to include heavier penalties if the guilty parties had also violated racial boundaries. In tracing Virginia legislative history (which is typical of the South), one finds an unswerving preoccupation with preserving those boundaries. A law enacted in 1787 declared that "every person who shall have one-fourth part or more of Negro blood shall be deemed a mulatto." There the color line held until 1910 when the state legislature, responding to increasing intermarriage between whites and blacks, declared that any person whose ancestry was one-sixteenth Negro was of that race.[4] Many Americans feared that dilution of the ancestral stock by mulattoes and blacks threatened the nation's future. According to one authority, between 1890 and 1910 the "colored" population increased by 81 percent, while the Negro population increased by only 22.7 percent.[5]

In Virginia the legislature responded by passing legislation titled "An Act to Preserve Racial Integrity."[6] The key feature of this law, the most powerful legal obstacle to interracial marriage erected since the Civil War, was to define a "white" person as one "who has no trace whatsoever of any blood other than Caucasian." Officials charged with issuing marriage licenses were ordered not to do so until they had "reasonable assurance that the statements as to color of both man and woman are correct." Existing interracial marriages were declared void regardless of the state in which they had been licensed, and interracial cohabitation was declared a crime. There was one exception to the antimiscegenation policy. The "Pocahontas exception," written in deference to the large number of persons who claimed to be descendants of Pocahontas and John Rolfe, permitted a white to marry "a person with one-sixteenth or less of the blood of an American Indian." At least two other states, Georgia and Alabama, followed Virginia's lead and defined as white only those persons whose genealogy was untainted.[7]

In Virginia the task of implementing the new antimiscegenation statute fell on the shoulders of the state registrar of vital statistics. Walter Ashby Plecker, a physician who earned his medical degree at the University of Maryland in 1885, had occupied the registrar's chair since 1912. Although he practiced medicine for many years in Hampton, Virginia, Plecker had been interested in public health since early in his career. By 1924 he had published a number of papers on issues in public health and eugenics, and had earned an entry in *Who's Who in American Medicine*.[8]

Plecker was deeply committed to enforcing the antimiscegenation measure. In February 1928, his battle to maintain "racial integrity" came to the attention of Laughlin. Their correspondence grew out of a letter that Dr. Plecker had written to Madison Grant, a wealthy New Yorker and a member of the inner circle of eugenicists. Plecker was lobbying for passage of a bill that would instruct the Census Bureau to abstract and publish the names of the heads of families as listed in each federal census since 1800. He thought that these data would help to verify the racial history of families, thus allowing him to identify persons trying to pass as white. He wrote to enlist Grant's support; Grant passed the letter to Laughlin, who wrote to learn more about the Virginia law.[9]

In reply, Plecker explained the Pocahontas exception and complained that it had created a loophole for "remnants of our so-called Indians who have in reality lost their identity by mixture with Negroes" to sneak across the color line. To deal with this problem Plecker had affixed a "warning" to birth and death certificates and marriage licenses that the Bureau of Vital Statistics would reclassify as "colored" any person either of whose parents had been classified as "Indian, Mixed Indian, Mixed, Melungeum, Issue, Free Issue, or other similar non-white terms."[10]

This letter excited Laughlin's interest in racial integrity laws, and he asked Plecker how other states dealt with this issue. Plecker sent him a list of current miscegenation statutes, and noted: "There is a disgracefully long list of states permitting the free intermarriage between whites and blacks. That is in reality the big problem as there is less tendency to intermarriage where there is any law at all forbidding intermarriage between the races, even though it be imperfect. A considerable number of our Virginia mixed breeds had migrated to Pennsylvania, New York and other northern states, I believe primarily to evade our marriage law."[11]

In his determination to deny white status to any Indian who had any Negro ancestry, Plecker even lobbied the Indian Office in Washington, D.C., to alter its definition of an Indian ("anyone with any Indian blood").[12] He was convinced that because persons living on a reservation in King William County, Virginia, had as much or more Negro as Indian blood, they should be considered colored, not Indian. The Indian Office did not pursue his suggestion. Seeing himself as a leader of a hopelessly outnumbered army, Plecker was, nevertheless, proud that his office would be able to save "young women, perhaps, from being misled into marrying mulattos under the guise of Indians."[13]

In 1930, after years of effort, Plecker convinced the Virginia legislature to amend its race law so that "Every person in whom there is ascertainable any Negro blood shall be deemed a colored person." This gave Plecker the power to redefine the racial status of the "mixed" breeds that had been attending white schools, and to banish the near-whites of Negro extraction to black schools. He was especially interested in reclassifying the "Mongrel Virginians," a group of perhaps one thousand near-white "mixed breeds" who had organized to fight the new law.[14]

Plecker's last known letter to Laughlin illustrates his crudely simple-minded understanding of the genetics of racial differences, and his virulent prejudice. He wrote, "I would feel somewhat easier about the matter if I thought that these near-whites would not produce children with negroid characteristics. I have never felt justified in believing that in some instances the children of mulattos are really white under Mendel's Law. At least I do not feel satisfied that we can know in an individual case that such is the fact."[15] Plecker's fear that a white-skinned descendant of a Negro could bear children with brown skin color was widely held at the time. Ironically, studies of black-white intermarriages in Jamaica conducted by Davenport two decades earlier had demonstrated that an "extracted white" would not bear a black child.[16]

Although many ardent proponents of eugenic sterilization believed that it would reduce the prevalence of crime, most early twentieth-century American criminologists flatly rejected this neo-Lombrosian thesis. For example, in his book, *Criminology* (1918), Maurice Parmelee asserted that Lombroso was "rather ignorant of the modern science of biology, and especially of the theory of heredity." Parmelee argued that what Lombroso had called "atavistic" traits were in reality examples of arrested development caused by an inhospitable environment. He admitted that hereditary factors sometimes figured in criminal conduct, but overall, he saw little value in sterilization as a means of reducing crime.[17]

Six years later, when Edwin Sutherland, a criminologist working at the University of Illinois, published his textbook, the vestiges of Lombrosian thought were sparse indeed. Sutherland wrote that "criminality as such cannot be inherited. If any trait is inherited which predisposes to crime, we do not know what it is. Even in the case of the feeble-minded and insane, it is not clear that their abnormalities are inherited, in the strict sense of the word, in a very large proportion of cases and, in addition, it is not clear that people with such difficulties are more prone to commit crimes than other people." Sutherland concluded that there was "no evidence that criminality would be reduced appreciably" by sterilization laws.[18]

Some contemporary journalists, however, advanced a more titillating view. For example, during 1924 and 1925 French Strother, editor of *World's Work,* a popular tabloid, wrote five articles on the biological basis of crime. These pieces illustrate how eugenics was portrayed for the lay reader. One article, "The Cause of Crime: Defective Brain," was a profile of Harry Olson's work as chief justice of the Chicago Municipal Court. Strother quoted Olson as asserting that "practically all criminals are mentally abnormal."[19] In 1914, convinced that it was time to use scientific methods in the service of crime prevention, Olson had founded the Psychopathic Laboratory. He instructed its director, Dr. William Hickson, a psychometrician, to develop "tests of character" to identify criminals. A decade later Strother reported that Hickson had discovered that dementia praecox (schizophrenia) was the cause of nearly all crimes, a finding that he promised would revolutionize criminology. Hickson's conclusions supplied Judge Olson, a staunch eugenicist, with exactly the mechanistic view of aberrant behavior that he sought. On returning from a tour of European psychology laboratories, Hickson reported to Olson that he had learned a new method of screening for criminal tendencies. He was convinced that nine out of ten criminals were mentally abnormal, and that he could identify more precisely the specific types of defects that led to crime. He suggested to reporters that the Chicago Police should round up the city's one hundred toughest characters and that those found by Psychopathic Laboratory tests to be abnormal should be committed *before* they harmed society.[20]

Another of Strother's articles, "The Cure for Crime," was a strident argument to "stop the breeding of mental defectives" as quickly as possible.[21] A third, which purported to be a primer on heredity, illustrated Mendelian inheritance by discussing the gene for Jewish facial appearance. Analyzing "all possible Jewish-Gentile crosses," Strother advised his readers that "all children of a Jew and a Gentile will look like Gentiles, that if a pure Gentile marries a half-Jew, all the children will look like Gentiles, and that if a half-Jew marries a half-Jew, one child of every four will look like a Jew and the other three will look like Gentiles."[22] Unfortunately, more people probably read Strother's article in one week than read genetics textbooks in an entire year.

The tireless efforts of a few prominent eugenicists like Judge Olson, who oversaw the work of thirty-six other judges, helped to keep pro-sterilization arguments viable during the years just after defeats in the courts. Olson flatly condemned the view in academic criminology circles that there was no persuasive evidence for the heritability of criminal tendencies. In his 1925 presidential address to the Eugenic Research Association, he asserted: "Crime prevention, finally, is seen to be the weeding out of defective stocks, and it is the first step in the eugenics program."[23]

Eugenics Societies

As Americans grew more discontented with the huge influx of immigrants in the postwar years, many people became interested in the problem of racial vigor. In dozens of towns across America, small groups of citizens organized to ponder this and other eugenic questions. Two of these organizations, the American Eugenics Society and the Human Betterment Foundation, attained some prominence. Although it is difficult to assess their impact on sterilization policy, there is no doubt that they published pamphlets, provided speakers, and worked assiduously to keep eugenics proposals, especially sterilization, alive as newsworthy topics.

Although the American Eugenics Society was not incorporated until 1926, it was started shortly after the Second International Congress of Eugenics met in New York City in September 1921. If the First International Eugenics Congress, which had convened in London in 1912, reflected the eugenic thinking in Great Britain, the New York City meeting showed that a group of committed eugenicists had emerged in the United States. Dr. Henry Fairfield Osborn, president of the American Museum of

Natural History, was chosen by his American colleagues as president of the Second International Congress, Madison Grant was elected treasurer, and the tireless Laughlin worked as chairman of the Exhibits Committee. After the congress closed, several prominent Americans, wanting to do more than maintain a committee affiliated with the London-based International Commission on Eugenics, formed the Eugenics Society of the United States of America.

By March 1923 this New York–based group, which changed its name to the American Eugenics Society (AES) in 1924, was sufficiently cohesive to be lobbying in Albany against legislation that it felt would have dysgenic effects. With strong support from the New York Charities Aid Association (an organization abhorred by hard-core eugenicists), two New York legislators had introduced a bill providing special educational assistance for "retarded" children (defined as those who were learning at a level that was three or more years below that expected for their age). The Austin-Cole Bill proposed providing state funds to stimulate the schools to hire more teachers to work in special education. A memorandum prepared by Laughlin for the AES about this bill described the proposed program as unequivocally "anti-eugenic," siphoning tax dollars that would be better spent on the gifted. He suggested lobbying to amend the law so that the retarded children could be sterilized. "Otherwise," he feared, "the education of the defective will bolster him or her up to the reproductive period and will make it more possible for him or her to become a parent than would be possible if he or she were less well trained." Despite the efforts of the AES, the bill became law.[24]

In the mid-twenties Irving Fisher, a professor of public policy at Yale, was the driving force behind the AES, which then maintained its headquarters in New Haven. Fisher enlisted a zealous but unsophisticated eugenicist named Leon Whitney to be the society's secretary. Whitney, a wealthy farmer and an avid dog breeder, had undergone an almost mystical conversion to eugenics, giving up his comfortable country life to plunge into a new career. In 1928 he published *The Basis of Breeding* (dedicated to Laughlin), a volume intended to educate laypersons about genetics. One key eugenics activity that Whitney extolled in his book was to sponsor "fitter family" contests. These contests frequently took place at fairs in the Midwest: judges reviewed human pedigrees to determine the most eugenically positive families, just as the best cattle, chickens, and pigs competed for blue ribbons.[25] He also helped the AES to construct a "Eugenics Catechism," a pamphlet of questions and answers about eugenics, and to launch the publication of a periodical called *Eugenics*.

During the Depression, when many of its leaders suffered heavy financial losses, the activities of the AES were greatly curtailed. By 1934 the society was broke, and Henry Perkins, a professor at the University of Vermont who was serving as its president, resigned in midterm. Ellsworth Huntington, a Yale political geographer, agreed to take the presidency of the group.[26] During Huntington's tenure (1934-38), Frederick Osborn, a wealthy relative of Henry Fairfield Osborn, used his financial clout to become the dominant force in the AES.

Both Huntington and Osborn agreed that in its early years the AES had focused too much on "negative" eugenic policies such as sterilization. They developed a grand plan encompassing public health, education, and birth control that would give "positive" eugenics a broadly based place in American life. Correctly sensing that this would be politically more palatable, they moved quickly to make AES activities appeal to the mainstream. Fisher, a utopian thinker, led the drive to rename the society. He wanted to eliminate the word *eugenics* and rename the organization the Society for Constructive Philanthropy, but he did not succeed.[27]

During the mid-1930s, Huntington and his colleagues worked assiduously to build bridges to other public welfare groups, and they met with some success. Perhaps their biggest victory was the publication of *Tomorrow's Children*, Huntington's far-sighted and provocative speculation on the potential rewards to be reaped from positive eugenics. Published by Wiley late in 1935, the book was well-reviewed and sold a respectable two thousand copies during its first year.[28] Between 1936 and 1938 membership in the AES doubled, a development that Huntington directly attributed to the society's more moderate image.[29]

These changes were opposed by a more radical wing, still centered at Cold Spring Harbor. In 1937, for example, Davenport declined to attend an advisory committee meeting, charging that the AES had adopted an orientation that attributed too much to the environment.[30] This split was exactly what Osborn wanted. In May 1938 he candidly wrote to Huntington, "I feel strongly, and believe you fully agree, that we ought not to tie our selves in with Laughlin and Davenport or the Record Office crowd."[31]

The years 1938-39 were the high-water mark for the new AES. In May 1938 S. J. Holmes, a renowned geneticist at Berkeley, accepted Huntington's invitation to succeed him as president.[32] In 1939 Waldeman Kaempffert, the science editor of the *New York Times* and a man who abhorred Laughlin's views, acknowledged that the AES had made the transition away from negative eugenics to a more acceptable line.[33] But just as its fortunes looked good, the AES was again buffeted by world affairs. With the onset of war in Europe, many of its leaders were drawn to Washington. Osborn took on a series of government posts that limited his role in the AES for the next decade. After World War II the organization again altered its goals, took on a new name (the Human Betterment Association), and devoted its energies to the question of world population control.

The second most influential eugenics society in the United States was the Human Betterment Foundation, the pet project of Ezra S. Gosney, a self-made millionaire who lived in Pasadena, California. Gosney became interested in eugenics late in his colorful career. Born in 1855 in Kenton County, Kentucky, he was educated at Richmond College in Missouri and earned a law degree at Washington University. He quickly established a good law practice (his main client was a railroad), but a severe illness redirected his life. About 1890 he settled in Flagstaff, Arizona, where he became deeply involved in the bitter struggle over grazing rights between cattlemen and sheep ranchers. He organized the Arizona Woolgrowers Association, which he served as president for ten years, and he started a successful bank. In 1905 Gosney, now quite wealthy, retired to Pasadena, where he became a leading civic figure, and he launched yet another com mercial venture. Seeing a market for citrus fruit, he developed one of California's largest lemon groves. It was about this time that he began to emerge as a philanthropist with a special interest in education. He con tributed half the funds needed to build the Polytechnic Elementary School, still one of America's leading private preparatory schools, and was very generous with scholarship money for Pasadena's Boy Scouts.[34]

Gosney first learned of the eugenics movement from a newspaper article that announced the opening of the Eugenics Record Office in Cold Spring Harbor in 1910. He wrote to Charles Davenport to learn more, and his interest soon became advocacy. By 1920, Gosney had become convinced that the crucial undertaking in eugenics would be to educate young people about the importance of mate selection. But despite his offers of financial support, he was unable to persuade any university to sponsor his unique educational plan. Thwarted in his first effort, Gosney turned his attention to the study of negative eugenics. He decided to analyze the history of sterilization in California. In 1926 Gosney organized a council of advisers, including Dr. J. H. McBride, a member of the state Commission on Immigration and Housing, and Paul Popenoe, a sociologist who edited the *Journal of Heredity*, to begin a detailed examination of how sterilization of thousands of California's defectives had affected the state. During this period his interest became a conviction, and in 1929 he created the Human Betterment Foundation (HBF), a nonprofit corporation intended to foster eugenics.

From the inception of the California sterilization study Gosney turned to Laughlin for advice.[35] Laughlin provided him with copies of the forms that he used to record and store eugenic data at the ERO and urged him to visit the state hospitals, advice probably given because Laughlin knew the frightening impact that large numbers of poorly housed feeble-minded persons could have on an inexperienced person. A few weeks later Gosney wrote Laughlin that McBride and Popenoe were visiting institutions around the state and that he was gathering the support of physicians and government officials for undertaking a much larger study of sterilization.[36] In reply, Laughlin sent the names and addresses of fifty-two persons whom he knew had been released from California hospitals after being sterilized so that Gosney could conduct a follow-up investigation on the long-term effects of vasectomy.[37]

In March of 1926 Gosney and Laughlin formally agreed to collaborate. From Gosney's perspective, at least, there was ample reason to do so: "It appears to me that there will be great value in having two independent and parallel studies of this topic. The whole project of sterilization is continually under attack, and is certain to be attacked still more vehemently if we proceed with an educational campaign on its behalf. To meet these attacks, we will need all the ammunition available, and it seems unquestionable that a single investigation would be less effective than a double investigation."[38]

By May 1927 Gosney had assembled an impressive list of consultants to the sterilization study. They included David Starr Jordan, chancellor of Stanford University, Lewis Terman, the nation's most prominent psychometrician, and S. J. Holmes, the Berkeley geneticist. Over the next few months the HBF consultants approved eighteen reports on the medical, psychological, economic, and legal dimensions of California's long-running (1909-27) sterilization program. Collectively these reports, all of which were published during the next three years, constituted the first comprehensive "proof" that sterilization was cost-effective and posed no significant medical harm to the institutionalized persons at whom it was aimed. Popenoe, who wrote many of the papers, reassured readers that the data revealed no evidence of discrimination because of race or ethnicity, and that two-thirds of those paroled after sterilization did "reasonably well" outside of the institutions. By 1928 his work was sufficiently well regarded that he was invited to address the annual meeting of the American Bar Association on the topic of sterilization and criminality.[39] *Sterilization for Human Betterment,* published by Gosney and Popenoe in 1929, was the first comprehensive discussion of sterilization aimed at the lay reader. They argued that under a scientifically applied sterilization program, "the number of mentally defective persons in the community could be reduced by perhaps as much as half in three or four generations."[40]

In 1930 the HBF began to conduct an annual survey of state sterilization programs. Like Dr. Sharp before World War I and Harry Laughlin in the 1920s, during the 1930s Edward Gosney and Paul Popenoe were the chief propagandists for and scorekeepers of eugenic sterilization in America. For example, in 1935 the HBF mailed over forty thousand pamphlets containing their sterilization survey results to professors at 436 colleges in every state and several foreign countries. During 1935, Gosney even convinced Harry Chandler, publisher of the *Los Angeles Times,* to run a column, "Social Eugenics," in the paper's Sunday magazine.[41]

By the late 1920s Gosney's name had begun to appear on the letterheads of the various eastern eugenics groups. In 1932 he was invited to speak at the Third International Congress on Eugenics in New York City. He must have regarded this as a signal honor, for despite his age and poor health, he took the long train ride across America. His speech at this last great gathering of eugenicists rejected the belief that segregation or involuntary contraception could effectively limit reproduction by defectives. He was convinced that any technique other than sterilization would result in the births of many more defective persons. The HBF was quite active until Gosney's death in 1942, when it too ceased to exist.

Although they were not as visible as the AES or as active as the Human Betterment Foundation, a few smaller eugenics groups probably had some influence on public attitudes in their states. The Brush Foundation is a good example. Charles Francis Brush was the quintessential successful American. Born in Ohio in 1849, he displayed an early interest in magnets and batteries, which blossomed into a magnificent career. After taking an engineering degree at the University of Michigan in 1869, he moved to Cleveland. There in 1877 he perfected an arc light which became the first system used for lighting Cleveland's streets. The Brush Electric Company profited greatly from the earnings on more than fifty patents that were awarded to its founder. By 1891, Brush, who had become a multimillionaire and a bank president, turned to philanthropy. In the early 1920s he became fascinated with eugenics, and in 1928 he established the Charles F. Brush Foundation for the Betterment of the Human Race. He endowed his new project with the princely sum of $500,000.[42]

Among the Brush Foundation's first projects was the support of the Race Betterment Conference convened by the Ohio Race Betterment Association in Dayton on October 10, 1929. Many prominent Ohio academicians, including Arthur Morgan, president of Antioch College, joined with the superintendents of the state's asylums and with leaders of the Brush Foundation to discuss eugenics. Interestingly, as the conference opened Brooks Shepherd, a foundation trustee, was careful to state that "we are not a branch of the American Eugenics Society." He steered a middle course, acknowledging that some eugenic claims were not well founded, "although some of them certainly are." As for sterilization, Shepherd was uncertain as to whether it or institutional segregation was the better choice. He urged that there be more scientific research in eugenics.[43]

At the same conference, Dr. William Pritchard, superintendent of the Columbus State Hospital, vehemently advocated a sterilization law. Noting that there were twenty-one thousand residents of the state's hospitals and eleven thousand prison inmates, he estimated that for at least half there was no hope of "recovery." Describing "complete and permanent segregation of all of the unfit" as physically and fiscally impossible, Pritchard stated that many feeble-minded and epileptic persons might be released "if the tendency toward sexual excesses, and consequent reproduction, could be curbed." He pleaded for support of a sterilization bill then languishing in the legislature.[44]

During 1930 a number of the key figures at the Race Betterment Conference did become deeply involved in a lobbying effort on behalf of a sterilization bill. The Ohio Race Betterment Association helped lead the lobbying effort, but it ran into heavy opposition. For example, R. E. Miles, director of the Ohio Institute, wrote a lengthy critique of involuntary sterilization based on arguments made by geneticist H. S. Jennings in *The Biological Basis of Human Nature.*[45]

Looking for ammunition with which to refute Jennings's position, Jerome Fisher, a Cleveland attorney who was chairman of the Ohio Race Betterment Association, wrote to Laughlin. Laughlin responded with a sympathetic letter, copies of several of his articles about sterilization laws, and a tightly argued six-page essay, "Answer to Jennings in Reference to Futility of Eugenical Sterilization."[46] Fisher used this material to counterattack, but the proponents of sterilization failed to secure a law for Ohio.

In addition to Gosney and Brush, several other wealthy men started societies or foundations intended to support the eugenics movement. The fate met by the J. Ewing Mears Fund indicates that sterilization was strongly opposed in at least some academic quarters. Dr. Mears, a prominent Philadelphia urologist and a staunch advocate of sterilization, had lobbied hard on behalf of the 1905 Pennsylvania bill that the governor had vetoed. When he died in 1919, Mears left his estate to his sister, stipulating that the legacy pass to Harvard University upon her death. The bequest required that eugenics "shall be taught in all its branches, notably that branch relat-

ing to the treatment of the defective and criminal classes by surgical procedures." In May 1927, at the height of the pro-sterilization movement,
Harvard rejected this substantial gift (sixty thousand dollars) because ac-
ceptance would be construed as approval of involuntary sterilization.[47]

Laughlin closely followed the legal battle that ensued as relatives and
various medical schools in Philadelphia vied for the money. In January
1930 the Supreme Court of Pennsylvania awarded the Mears Fund to
Jefferson Medical College and permitted more latitude in its use than had
been provided by the will.[48] A year later Laughlin, writing in his capacity
as editor of *Eugenical News,* asked how the money was being spent. The
dean replied that the plan would be to explore "broad problems of heredity," not just "contraceptive measures."[49] Reflecting on the loss of this
money from the coffers of the pro-sterilization forces, Laughlin scribbled
a note: "Wouldn't this make a minister strike his father? At any rate the
heirs didn't get it and eugenics did."

One of the most colorful and zealous (if ineffective) eugenicists of the
1930s was a Kansas City businessman named J. H. Pile. In 1938, extremely
concerned by the sharply declining birth rate that the Depression fostered,
Pile set up the Eugenic Babies Foundation. It was intended to increase
reproduction by women "above the average in intellect" and to deny parenthood to "chronic paupers, confirmed criminals, feeble-minded and
insane persons." Pile, who hoped for an endowment of one hundred million dollars, launched a campaign to enlist the United States Chamber of
Commerce and the various eugenics societies in his cause. He frequently
wrote to the AES. However, Huntington and Osborn eschewed involve-
ment with radical groups, and they decided to "steer clear of Mr.
Pile."[50] Pile's utopian fantasy should not, however, be dismissed too quickly. While his proposals were ridiculed in the United States, German officials
were initiating *Lebensborn,* a program that involved kidnapping eugenically desirable children from Poland and elsewhere, and setting up special
homes where the sturdiest German girls were urged to become pregnant by
select German soldiers and bear their "superior" babies.[51]

In 1939 the AES was courted by another would-be eugenic philanthropist. After his graduation from Princeton at the turn of the century,
James G. Eddy made a fortune in the lumber industry. He later founded the
Institute for Forest Genetics, which contributed substantially to that field
and earned the support of the Carnegie Institute. In 1938 Eddy approached
Laughlin, offering to support a human heredity clinic that would alert
couples to the risk of bearing defective babies. Laughlin carried the plan to
the directors of the Carnegie Institute (a mistake, since he was in disfavor),
who rejected it as being too removed from basic research. Eddy then asked

if the AES would consider operating such a clinic for which he would provide one-half the first year's budget. Although Osborn admired Eddy, he and Huntington agreed that a "marriage reference bureau" was too limited an operation for the AES.[52] Just a few years later the Dight Institute at the University of Minnesota started a similar clinic that was perhaps the nation's first genetic counseling center.

Although the 1930s saw a general shift of emphasis toward programs that enhanced principles of positive eugenics, some groups continued to push for sterilization. The mandate of the Sterilization League of New Jersey (to be discussed more fully in Chapter 7), which began in Princeton in 1934, was to put "a check on the reproduction of defectives." The president was T. L. Zimmerman, a former judge of the Juvenile and Domestic Relations Court in Bergen County. For nearly a decade the league lobbied arduously but unsuccessfully for a sterilization law. Despite repeated legislative defeats at home, the league was a tireless propagandist for eugenic sterilization.

The Second Wave of Sterilization Laws

After a peak in 1913, when five new states adopted sterilization laws, legislative activity slowed significantly. From 1918 until the end of 1922, only Washington was added to the ranks, while seven other state laws were invalidated. But in 1923 there was a resurgence of legislative activity, and eugenic sterilization laws were enacted in Oregon, Montana, Delaware, and Michigan. Virginia adopted a sterilization law the following year, and in 1925 the legislative floodgates opened. Nine state legislatures passed bills, and seven were enacted (two were vetoed). Of these Idaho, Utah, Minnesota, and Maine enacted their first eugenic sterilization laws. At the end of 1925, enabling legislation to support sterilization programs was law in seventeen states.

Advocates had learned from the mistakes made in earlier legislative efforts. For example, after carefully analyzing the constitutional infirmities of the early laws, Laughlin drafted a model eugenic sterilization bill that purported to safeguard the procedural rights of the persons to whom it might be applied, and that satisfied the Equal Protection Clause. The bill required the state eugenicist to conduct surveys to identify persons who were "potential parents of socially inadequate offspring." Such surveys would canvass the entire population, not merely the residents of state institutions, without regard to "personality, sex, age, marital condition, race or possessions." If the state eugenicist determined that an individual was a potential parent of socially inadequate offspring and a candidate for

involuntary sterilization, the statute required a hearing, followed automatically by a jury trial and the right of appeal. Although no state enacted
the precise text of Laughlin's bill (a draft of which was approved by the
American Bar Association Committee on Sterilization), many of its features
were incorporated into new bills. The phrase "potential parent of socially
inadequate offspring" was widely copied.[53]

What was the attitude of state officials in regard to implementing these
new statutes? An unpublished manuscript, entitled "Sterilization of the
Unfit Degenerates," which contains the results of a survey of state officials
conducted in 1925 by the Rhode Island State Library, sheds some light on
this question.[54] For example, the Connecticut state librarian responded
that he found no evidence of eugenic sterilizations performed in that state's
institutions during the prior ten years.[55]

The executive director of the Delaware Board of Charities, J. Hall
Anderson, reported that without benefit of legislation (but with the consent
of the families), he had authorized the sterilization of four patients. Anderson strongly advocated a broad sterilization law to cover "cases outside
of Institutions," but noted that "in the present state of political opinion it
would probably be impossible to get the Legislature to sanction such a
drastic measure." This comment was made just when many legislatures
were passing compulsory sterilization laws, suggesting that public opinion
drew the line firmly at the institution's portals.[56]

Officials in Kansas, a state that adopted a very aggressive sterilization
policy in the mid-1920s, worried that the public might be offended by
overzealous application of the law. Charles S. Huffman, a member of the
Board of Educational, Charitable and Correctional Institutions, noted that
"the larger number of protests come from those of the Catholic faith who
claim it is against their religious teachings to interfere with nature." Catholic opposition to sterilization became quite active during the mid-1930s.
Nevertheless, Kansas was one of the first states whose officials explicitly
adopted a policy of sterilizing "most all feeble-minded, institutionalized
women patients of the childbearing age."[57]

Just as they had in the past, opponents of involuntary sterilization laws
launched a constitutional attack on the flurry of new laws. The battle was
joined in two states, Michigan and Virginia. The Michigan law, which
contemplated sterilizing "idiots, imbeciles, and the feeble-minded, but not
the insane," was not limited to institutionalized persons. Shortly after an
order by the Wayne County Probate Court that one Willie Smith should be
sterilized by "vasectomy or X-ray," his guardian *ad litem* challenged the
law. On June 18, 1925, the Supreme Court of Michigan ruled that the
statute was "justified by the findings of Biological Science," and was "a

proper and reasonable exercise of the police power of the state." The high court also held that a section of the law that exempted from sterilization wealthy feeble-minded persons who could pay for the care of their children was a violation of the Equal Protection Clause. Nevertheless, the Michigan decision, the first by a state supreme court to uphold a eugenic sterilization law, was a major victory for the pro-sterilization forces.[58]

The constitutional challenge to the Virginia law, which was ultimately decided by the Supreme Court of the United States, had the largest impact on eugenic sterilization programs. Early in 1924 the Virginia legislature, noting that "heredity plays an important part in the transmission of insanity, idiocy, imbecility, epilepsy and crime," overwhelmingly passed an involuntary sterilization bill (the Senate voted 30-0; the House, 75-2). The law, which gave the superintendents of five state institutions the power to petition a special board for permission to sterilize those inmates whom they believed it would benefit, was signed by the governor on March 20, 1924.[59]

On January 23, 1924, an eighteen-year-old woman named Carrie E. Buck, the illegitimate daughter of an allegedly feeble-minded woman named Addie Emmet, who had been adopted by a Charlottesville family at the age of four, was committed to the State Colony for Epileptics and Feeble-Minded. Always a problem child, Carrie, who was said to have a mental age of nine and an I.Q. of about 50, had recently given birth to an illegitimate child who was also allegedly feeble-minded. Fearing that Carrie would bear more children in the State Colony, Dr. A. S. Priddy, the superintendent, petitioned for sterilization. Realizing that the law would eventually be challenged, state officials were eager to make this the test case. In searching for an expert witness, they asked the advice of Judge Olson, who recommended Harry Laughlin. Although he never saw the patient, on the basis of his review of her records Laughlin concluded that Carrie was part of the "shiftless, ignorant and worthless class of anti-social whites of the South." He noted that her sexual immorality was "a typical picture of the low-grade moron," and that the possibility of her feeble-mindedness being due to nonhereditary causes was "exceptionally remote."[60]

On September 10, 1924, the board approved the sterilization of Carrie Buck. A young attorney named R. G. Shelton was appointed as her guardian, and he immediately appealed to the Circuit Court of Amherst County, Virginia. The case was argued on November 18, 1924, and Laughlin's deposition was submitted into evidence. On April 13, 1925, Judge Bennet Gordon upheld the constitutionality of the law and ordered that Carrie be sterilized within ninety days. The record that the proponents of the law compiled was impressive. Besides the testimony of Laughlin, they secured the support of Dr. J. S. DeJarnett, superintendent of the largest state institution in Indiana, and Dr. Arthur Estabrook, a colleague of Laughlin's at Cold Spring Harbor who specialized in pedigree analysis and who had worked as a eugenics adviser to the state of Indiana. Shelton secured *no* experts to testify on Carrie Buck's behalf. In upholding the decision of the local court, the Virginia Supreme Court of Appeals rejected Carrie's argument that the law violated the Equal Protection Clause of the Constitution. Judge Jesse P. West ruled that the statute constituted a reasonable kind of class legislation that was intended to *benefit* the persons who would be sterilized. The decision was affirmed without dissent.[61]

On February 6, 1926, Carrie Buck appealed to the United States Supreme Court. Although the highest court had refused to hear arguments on the validity of sterilization laws in the past, this time it permitted the appeal, and the case was argued in the autumn. In his brief, Shelton presciently warned that if the law was upheld, "A reign of doctors will be inaugurated and in the name of science new classes will be added, even races may be brought within the scope of such a regulation and the worst forms of tyranny practiced." This is, of course, a capsule summary of Nazi eugenics.[62]

On May 2, 1927, by vote of 8 to 1, the Supreme Court upheld the Virginia involuntary sterilization law. Justice Oliver Wendell Holmes, eighty-six years old at the time, wrote the brief majority opinion. In now famous words, Holmes asserted: "It is better for all the world, if instead of waiting to execute degenerate offspring for crime, or to let them starve for their imbecility, society can prevent those who are manifestly unfit from continuing their kind. The principle that sustains compulsory vaccination is broad enough to cover cutting the Fallopian tubes."[63]

Dismissing the objection that the Virginia statute violated the Equal Protection Clause by treating institutionalized persons differently from those not in institutions as "the last resort of constitutional arguments," Holmes, whose published letters strongly suggest that he was a eugenicist,[64] opened the doors to eugenic sterilization in the United States. Justice Butler, the only dissenter, did not file an opinion. Although the resurgence of sterilization laws had been under way for four years when *Buck v. Bell* was decided, the Supreme Court ruling greatly boosted the pace at which sterilization programs were enacted and implemented. During the next few years the number of states with sterilization laws jumped from seventeen to thirty, and the number of sterilizations performed on institutionalized persons rose substantially. The subsequent fifteen years (1927-42) were a triumphant period for those who embraced hereditarian hopes for social progress.

7 · Sterilization Data

I wrote and delivered a decision upholding the constitutionality of a state law for sterilizing imbeciles the other day—and felt I was getting near to the first principle of real reform.
—Oliver Wendell Holmes, Jr., 1927

A consumer health group asserted yesterday that states are still sterilizing poor Medicaid recipients without properly obtaining their consent and even when they are younger than 21.
—*Boston Globe,* July 27, 1981

The decision of the United States Supreme Court to uphold Virginia's involuntary sterilization law signaled a new era in eugenics. In 1927 Indiana and North Dakota adopted sterilization laws, and in 1928 Mississippi followed suit. During 1929 nine other states enacted sterilization laws. Only three of these laws were the first in their respective states (Arizona, Maine, and West Virginia), but the extensive revisions of existing statutes indicate that eugenic sterilization was a major legislative topic that year. All the laws enacted between 1927 and 1930 included procedural safeguards comparable to those in the Virginia law that had been upheld by the Supreme Court. Eugenicists could rest assured that unlike the situation a decade earlier, the laws would survive constitutional attack. During the next five years (1930-34), eugenic sterilization bills continued to meet with substantial success. In 1931 sterilization bills were introduced in ten states and became law in five, raising the number of states with enabling statutes to twenty-eight.[1]

Energized by *Buck v. Bell* and hoping to secure a law in every state, the AES Committee on Legislation redoubled its efforts. But in some states there was much opposition. The AES chose William C. Palmer to lead a lobbying campaign that focused on New Jersey and Kentucky. Despite much effort, the proponents of sterilization failed in both states. Defeat in

New Jersey, where support by the League of Women Voters and the Federation of Women's Clubs had made prospects look good, was especially bitter. Roswell Johnson, editor of the *Eugenics* newsletter, attributed the loss to "religious prejudice," a not too veiled reference to the Catholic church, a perennial adversary. In Kentucky defeat was largely caused by the submission of a poorly drafted bill that proposed sterilizing all habitual criminals. One senator remarked that if such a law had been passed forty years earlier, "there would not be so many fools here [in the Senate] now." Another lawmaker offered an amendment that all Republicans be sterilized. The bill drowned in a tidal wave of guffaws.[2]

Physician Advocates

Influential as it was, *Buck v. Bell* does not by itself explain why during the late 1920s and the early 1930s so many legislatures were favorably disposed toward eugenic sterilization. Another important factor is that eugenicists successfully elicited support from physician groups. After Dr. Robert Dickinson, a leading gynecologist and a member of the Committee on Maternal Health of the American Eugenics Society, lectured on sterilization at the annual meeting of the American Medical Association in 1928, he told fellow AES members that the physicians had shown "great interest" in his data on eugenic sterilization.[3] In 1929, the American Association for the Study of the Feeble-Minded (the descendant of the AMO and a group that included many physicians) held its fifty-third annual meeting in Atlanta. According to Dr. Harry W. Crane, a North Carolina psychologist, the association agreed that it was "absolutely impossible to cope with the problem of feeble-mindedness without judicious use of sterilization."[4] Dr. Harvey M. Watkins, superintendent of the State School in Polk, Pennsylvania, surveyed the members of the American Association for the Study of the Feeble-Minded about current sterilization programs. Respondents answered his inquiry, "Do you approve of sterilization of the mentally defective?" with an overwhelmingly (227-16) affirmative vote. After analyzing the reasons why this view was held, Watkins noted that concern among physicians was shifting from the control of genetic disorders to reducing procreation by socially inadequate parents.[5]

During the decade after *Buck v. Bell* (1927-1936), approximately sixty medical articles, the vast majority favoring the practice, were published about sterilization. Regional journals, such as the *Virginia Medical Monthly,* frequently published pro-sterilization articles. But articles favoring sterilization of the mentally deficient also appeared in the prestigious pages of the *New England Journal of Medicine.*[6] These articles rarely examined the scientific underpinnings of the programs. Rather, they focused on the safety of the operation and its impact on the lives of the patients. During the years in which sterilization of institutionalized persons was most aggressively pursued, there were few systematic studies of the scientific validity of this policy.

One relatively large study, conducted by physicians at Elwyn, Pennsylvania, in 1931, was published too late to cause us to suspect that it influenced legislators. However, it is of interest because it followed up 270 patients who had been sterilized at Elwyn since the 1890s.[7] Given that Pennsylvania had never enacted a law permitting sterilizations, this is extraordinary. It suggests that the actual number of eugenic sterilizations carried out in the United States significantly exceeded those allowed by state law.

As they had during the first wave of legislation before World War I, a few physicians played key roles in stimulating the resurgence of the sterilization movement. The work of Dr. Charles Fremont Dight in Minnesota deserves special mention. Dight became involved in the eugenics movement in 1922 when he joined the Eugenics Research Association. In 1923 he became a charter member of the American Eugenics Society, and during that year he started the Minnesota Eugenics Society. In 1924, at the age of sixty-six, he began writing articles on sterilization, and he became extremely active in lobbying for a sterilization law in his home state. Minnesota adopted such a law in 1925 (by a vote of 86-37 in the House and 40-4 in the Senate), and Dight was given credit for its enactment.[8]

But Dight, a former Minneapolis alderman, was far from satisfied with the law, which was only applied to a few dozen institutionalized persons each year. During the 1930s he regularly sponsored radio broadcasts arguing that thousands of persons needed to be sterilized. At times he was almost fanatical in his effort to extend the law's reach. Although he never succeeded in his effort to sterilize large numbers of noninstitutionalized persons, Dight did win the support of some powerful state officials. For example, in 1927 Francis Kuhlman, a prominent psychologist who was the director of the Division of Research of the Minnesota Department of Public Institutions, spoke in favor of Dight's plan to extend sterilization to the "high-grade feeble-minded."[9] Another important ally was Dr. E. P. Lyon, a professor at the University of Minnesota School of Medicine, who lobbied vigorously to expand the sterilization program. By his death, Dight, who had stipulated that his estate should found an Institute of Human Genetics at the University of Minnesota, was a nationally known sterilization advocate.

The activities of Robert P. C. Wilson are typical of other dedicated physician advocates. Wilson, a psychiatrist, spent twenty-five years working at Missouri's School for the Feeble Minded and Epileptic, located in Marshall. In November 1933, Judge Daniel Taylor, a member of the Board of Managers of the State Eleemosynary Institutions, visited the school. Wilson seized the opportunity and spoke out strongly in favor of a eugenic sterilization plan. Judge Taylor, who was "totally upset" by seeing the "hopeless unfortunates," promised to introduce a sterilization bill at the next legislative session.[10] Encouraged by the support of Taylor and other officials who visited the hospital, and concerned by the steady growth in its patient population, Wilson embarked on a one-man statewide campaign for a sterilization bill. During 1936 he stumped the state, spoke often, and assiduously cultivated newspaper coverage.[11] Although he evoked considerable public discussion, Dr. Wilson was unable to push the bill he drafted through the Statehouse.

The editors of *Eugenics,* the monthly magazine intended to keep the public abreast of the movement's progress, regularly noted that physicians figured prominently in legislative efforts. For example, the 1929 West Virginia law, which easily passed both houses, was drafted by Dr. B. W. West, a physician in private practice.[12] In January 1931, Roswell Johnson, who wrote the "Legislation" column for *Eugenics,* surveyed the upcoming state legislative session and concluded that prospects for securing a new sterilization law were best in Georgia, where two physicians, Dr. Joseph P. Bowdoin of the State Board of Health and Dr. W. P. Pace, a member of the legislature and author of a proposed sterilization bill, were "ready to push it."[13]

A series of articles in the *Journal of Psycho-Asthenics,* the official publication of the American Association for the Study of the Feeble-Minded, regularly offered clinical justification for sterilization. Since the journal was regularly read by the directors of the sixty-three state institutions for the care of the feeble-minded that then existed in America (only four states—Arizona, Arkansas, Montana, and New Mexico—did not have at least one), such articles reached a critical audience. Naturally, in an era of severe economic constraints brought on by the Depression, the superintendents of these institutions (fifty-four were physicians) were interested in programs that seemed to enhance the lives of their patients while helping to control the size of their budgets.

A speech that Dr. Harvey M. Watkins, superintendent of the Polk State School in Pennsylvania, delivered to the association in 1930 illustrates this point. Acknowledging that clinical studies had "modified the extreme viewpoint of heredity as demonstrated in the Jukes and the Kallikaks," he nevertheless argued that there were the "greatest social reasons" to support sterilization. Interwoven with his assertions that the operation benefited the patients were blunt economic facts. In his words: "No state can afford to continue building institutions sufficiently large to take care of the problem of the mentally defective, which is being increasingly recognized daily. Some measure other than permanent custodial care must be and should be found." Watkins applauded the program in Sonoma, California, where all defective persons were sterilized before they were "allowed to leave the State Home." He saw sterilization as the key to successful parole and the only practical way to permit the institutions to help other patients waiting for admission. His views were strongly seconded by his colleagues.[14]

In 1934 Dr. L. Potter Harshman, a psychiatrist at the Fort Wayne State School in Indiana, investigated the level of support provided by state medical societies to proponents of eugenic sterilization. Of the forty-two societies that responded to his questionnaire, eighteen indicated that they had "officially" supported a sterilization program in their states. The House of Delegates of the American Medical Association reported that in 1928 it had considered the matter but had taken no action.

Dr. Harshman also conducted a detailed study of sterilization orders in Indiana. He asked eighty-eight judges and 447 physicians about their decisions to sterilize 465 feeble-minded patients in Indiana between 1931 and 1934. While the physicians had been virtually unanimous in approving the proposed sterilization of persons sent to them for evaluation, the judges were remarkable for the polarity of their views. Twenty-six judges approved every sterilization petition brought before them, twenty-four refused to order the sterilization of any patient, and thirty-four split their decisions. Harshman concluded that the fifty-four judges who invariably decided one way or the other must have had strong personal views about eugenic sterilization. A staunch advocate of sterilization of the feeble-minded, Harshman urged physicians to lecture about its benefits before county bar associations and law schools, no doubt hoping to influence reluctant judges.

Harshman's study, which he reported at the 1935 meeting of the AMO, elicited a number of comments that provide insight into the status of sterilization programs in various states. A New Hampshire physician seconded his call for education, asserting that "any Judge . . . would listen respectfully" to scientific proof of hereditary taint. But Dr. B. D. Whitten, superintendent of the State Training School in Clinton, South Carolina, confided that he had stopped lobbying for a sterilization law when he learned that legislators thought it would permit them to reduce the institutional budget. Dr. J. M. Murdoch, superintendent of the Minnesota School for the Feeble-Minded, reported that as was the case in California, he sterilized all those who were to be released from the institution. Finally, the superintendent of a school in Northville, Michigan, reported that performing just a few sterilizations had engulfed him in a local controversy.[15]

Sterilization was a major topic of the American Association for Mental Deficiency at its 1935 meeting. Most physicians thought that the children of mentally defective women inevitably required placement, and that all defective women in their reproductive years should be sterilized. Physicians from several states (Vermont, Minnesota, and Michigan) urged that, despite the existence of compulsory laws, it was imperative to seek the consent of the patient's family, but they seemed motivated as much by fear of political reprisals as by concerns for patient rights.[16]

The discussions about sterilization policy at the annual meetings of the American Association for Mental Deficiency during the 1930s show that a new set of concerns motivated eugenic thinking. Fears that immigrants from southern and eastern Europe would dilute and weaken American social stock had faded, and aberrant social behavior was no longer thought to be genetically determined. As experts became more convinced that a deprived early home life could cause severe developmental problems, eugenicists urged the case for sterilizing young, mildly retarded women, especially those who had already proven themselves to be "bad" mothers. This new policy was strongly reinforced by the economic constraints of the Depression. The budgets of state hospitals were shrinking while the waiting lists were growing. It is not surprising, then, that during the middle and late 1930s, the annual number of sterilizations performed in the United States reached new heights.

Sterilization Data: Proof of the Victory

Although the army of pro-sterilization advocates was never large, it seemed always to include a few officers who worked far beyond the call of duty. For fifty years people like Harvey Sharp, Harry Laughlin, and Edwin Gosney were instrumental in keeping pro-sterilization arguments in the public mind. They never tired of collecting data, issuing press releases, writing letters to editors, and producing and distributing pamphlets. One important aspect of their work was to tally the progress of eugenic sterilization in the various states. Each year from 1920 through 1963 some member of the inner circle of pro-sterilization advocates conducted a thorough survey of virtually all institutions in the United States where sterilizations were (or might be) conducted.

During the 1920s, Laughlin regularly published the results of his surveys in the *Eugenical News,* a small monthly periodical for which he provided much of the copy. About every four years (1922, 1926, 1929) he included these data in his book-length monographs on the status of sterilization programs. In the 1930s, Edwin Gosney, president of the Human Betterment Foundation in Pasadena, underwrote the cost of extremely thorough annual surveys. During the 1940s, Marion Olden, a zealous advocate of eugenic sterilization and secretary of the Sterilization League of New Jersey (which she helped launch in 1937), took on the task of continuing the annual surveys. Olden and her successors continued to compile and publish eugenic sterilization data until 1963.

Four decades of survey data, summary statistics that were frequently enriched by comments in the covering letters sent by the officials at the various institutions, provide a rich mash from which to distill conclusions about the course run by eugenic sterilization. Analysis of these reports permits one to draw a number of conclusions:

—Throughout much of this century (1907-63) many states conducted programs intended to achieve the involuntary sterilization of institutionalized persons.
—More than sixty thousand persons were sterilized under these laws.
—Sterilization programs were most active during the 1930s, but in several states major sterilization programs were active in the 1940s and 1950s.
—Over time there were major geographical shifts in the level of activity of sterilization programs. Until the early 1930s California was responsible for nearly half of the sterilizations performed on institutionalized persons in the United States. During the 1920s several Midwestern states also had vigorous programs. In the early 1930s several southern states became deeply committed to eugenic sterilization. In the 1950s Virginia and North Carolina operated the nation's most active programs.
—During the Depression there was a major change in the factors that most concerned those officials who were empowered to sterilize. They became less concerned with preventing the birth of children with genetic defects and more concerned with preventing parenthood in those individuals who were thought to be unable to care for children. The goal was to reduce new burdens on the public purse. This generated a dramatic change in who was sterilized.
—Beginning about 1930 there was a steady rise in the percentage of young women who were sterilized. In a few states *only* young

women were sterilized. From 1930 until the early 1960s sterilizations were performed on many more institutionalized women
than men.
—Revulsion over Germany's racist politics did little to curtail
American programs before or after World War II. Indeed, American advocates pointed to Germany to illustrate how an enlightened sterilization program might quickly reach its goals.
—During the 1940s there was a sharp decline in the number of institutionalized persons sterilized each year in the United States. It
was caused predominantly by the shortage of civilian physicians
during World War II.
—After the war there was a transient increase, but in most states
the number of eugenic sterilizations did not return to prewar levels.

The letters that superintendents of the state hospitals sent in reply to
the HBF annual questionnaire indicate the status of various programs and
the attitudes of those who were actually deciding who should be sterilized.
The dimensions of each program depended on the specifics of the enabling
legislation, how well the program was funded, and the extent to which
individual superintendents supported the plan. For example in 1933 a
Mississippi official complained that the state law was procedurally "so
technical that it is almost impossible to comply with."[17] A West Virginia
official complained that opponents had so amended the sterilization law
"as to practically annul it."[18] An Arizona official reported that he had not
launched a program because the government had not agreed to pay for
judicial and medical costs. Clearly, enactment of a law did not always
guarantee an active sterilization program.

In some states the programs depended directly on the political clout
of the superintendents. Some officials had little power to get funds. Others,
like W. D. Partlow, an Alabama physician in charge of the state hospital
system, used their connections to secure funds for large-scale programs. He
sterilized "all inmates dismissed from our School for Feeble-minded," 184
persons in two years.[19] In Indiana W. F. Dunham, general superintendent of
the Fort Wayne State School, reported that despite his great interest in
sterilizing "acquired cases of feeblemindedness for purely social and economic reasons," he did not think that he could influence the general public
to accept "sterilizing at random in the counties."[20]

In 1934 the HBF conducted a survey to determine whether and how
consent was obtained to permit the sterilization of a feeble-minded or
insane person. The results indicated that efforts to obtain proxy consent

from relatives varied widely, ranging from the appointment of a special guardian to argue against the operation to making no effort at all. In Nebraska, New Hampshire, and Wisconsin sterilizations were not performed without consent of an appropriate family member. In South Dakota consent received only perfunctory attention, being obtained "less than 50%" of the time.[21] In North Carolina an official reported that consent was not usually obtained, but that family members knew of the operations and objected infrequently.[22]

The cost of eugenic sterilizations, especially as more operations were performed upon women, was a pressing concern. In 1934 an Idaho official reported that only one female had been sterilized that year because the legislature had not appropriated funds.[23] In reply to the 1939 survey, an official at the Utah State Training School reported that there was a backlog of "91 cases," patients who would be sterilized as soon as the school's hospital had the necessary surgical facilities.[24]

Replies to the annual HBF surveys suggest that there were many clandestine operations and that its official tally significantly underestimated the number of sterilizations being performed on defective persons. The assistant attorney general of Maine declared, "I know very well that many more operations have been performed [than are reported] but I suppose we shall have to go by the records."[25] A probate judge in Michigan reported that he knew that at least 71 "illegal sterilizations" (performed on noninstitutionalized defectives) had occurred.[26] The commissioner of public welfare in Vermont wrote that he believed the number of eugenic sterilizations was underreported.[27]

How many institutionalized persons in the United States were legally sterilized from 1907 through 1941? As shown in table 4, despite the flurry of legislative activity before World War I, during the first decade there were only 1,422 operations performed in the entire nation. Of that number 1,077 were performed in California, 118 in Indiana, and 67 in Iowa. Yet, despite subsequent (1916-20) judicial decisions that overturned many sterilization laws, the number of operations performed each year steadily increased. During the three-year period from 1918 through 1920, there were 1,811 sterilizations, about one-half of which were performed in California. Coincident with *Buck v. Bell,* a substantial change occurred in the late 1920s. In 1925 officials reported that 322 institutionalized persons were sterilized. During 1928 and 1929 there were 2,362 sterilizations, more than triple the 1925 rate. This was due to the rapid increase in the number of states with sterilization laws. For example, before 1927 one could not legally sterilize a feeble-minded person in Virginia, but from 1927 through 1937 about 1,000 eugenic operations were performed there.

Table 4 Sterilizations of Institutionalized Persons in the United States, 1907-1941 (Cumulative Totals)

| Year | Cumulative | | | Single Year Totals |
	Total	Male	Female	
1941	38,087	15,780	22,307	2,209
1940	35,878	14,900	20,978	2,843
1939	33,035	13,731	19,304	2,345
1938	30,690	12,795	17,895	2,821
1937	27,869	11,628	16,241	2,466
1936	25,403	10,674	14,729	2,237
1935	23,166	9,841	13,325	3,103
1934	20,063			
1933				
1932	16,066	6,999	9,067	3,921
1931	12,145			
1930				
1929	10,877			2,362
1928				
1927	8,515	4,517	3,998	
1926				
1925	6,244			322
1924	5,922	3,167	2,755	
1923				
1922				
1921				
1920	3,233[a]			
1919				
1918				
1917	1,422[b]			
1916				
1915				
1914				
1913				
1912				
1911				
1910				
1909				
1908				
1907				

[a]Of this total, 2,016 persons (63 percent) were sterilized in California.
[b]As of March 1, 1918. Of this total, 1,077 persons (70 percent) were sterilized in California.

Perhaps the most significant finding from the HBF data is that between 1928 and 1932 there was a dramatic change in the gender of those persons who were sterilized. At the end of 1927, about 53 percent of all persons who had ever been legally sterilized in the United States were male. During the next five years, 5,069 females (67 percent) and 2,482 males (33 percent) were sterilized in institutions in the United States. This focus on sterilizing young women continued throughout the 1930s. From 1932 through 1934, sterilizations were performed on 4,258 women (60 percent) and 2,842 men (40 percent). This gender imbalance is not explained by sex differences in mental retardation. There was, in fact, a significant (at least ten percent) excess of affected males in most state schools for the retarded.

Institutional reports show that young women who were at most mildly retarded were often admitted for the sole purpose of being sterilized. Officials then discharged them, confident that they could not become pregnant and bear children destined to be wards of the state. This approach was first taken in Wisconsin. Its law was enacted in 1913, and a team of physicians was promptly appointed to trace the family histories of institutionalized patients. In the summer of 1915 the operations commenced, and Dr. John R. V. Lyman sterilized 22 male patients. The team then turned its attention to the women patients; in the summer of 1916, sterilizations were performed on 35 female patients in the Home for the Feeble-Minded.[28] During the next 16 years, 382 residents of Wisconsin institutions were sterilized, of whom 18 were male and 364 female.[29]

In Minnesota prior to July 1, 1926, only 21 sterilizations had been performed pursuant to state law. Over the next twelve years there were 1,280 sterilizations performed on 1,078 females and 202 males (table 5).[30] Similarly, in Virginia between 1927 and 1937, 609 women, but only 391 men, were sterilized. As a physician from a Virginia institution put it, after "the sterilization law was finally declared constitutional, there was a rush to sterilize as many patients as possible and as quickly as possible." This was the only way to ensure turnover in patients, for otherwise "the female patient had to be confined in the hospital during her child-bearing period."[31] A program of admission, prompt sterilization, and speedy discharge of mildly retarded young women was also pursued in New Hampshire, where, from 1928 through 1937, 364 women and 62 men were sterilized.[32] This gender disequilibrium is impressive when one considers that the vasectomy is a low-risk procedure, and that during the 1930s the tubal ligation constituted major abdominal surgery. At least three women residing in California institutions and two women in Virginia institutions died after undergoing involuntary sterilization.[33]

About 1929, the number of eugenic sterilizations performed each year

Table 5 Sterilizations of Institutionalized Persons in Minnesota, 1926-1938

Year	Total	Male	Female
1938	151	40	111
1937	189	44	145
1936	81	21	60
1935	140	28	112
1934	144	21	123
1933	93	6	87
1932	79	7	72
1931	75	8	67
1930	60	8	52
1929	68	6	62
1928	57	7	50
1927	90	4	86
1926	53	2	51
	1,280	202	1,078

Note: These data are abstracted from biennial reports of the State Board of Control of Minnesota, 1926-38.

upon institutionalized persons jumped. The consistency of this event across state lines suggests a real policy shift. For example, from 1925 to 1929 there were only 21 operations performed in South Dakota, but in the next six years 248 feeble-minded persons were sterilized.[34] In the first five years of its program, North Carolina sterilized 53 persons. But in 1934 (when a new law expanded the program's reach to the entire state population) sterilizations were performed on 61 persons, and in 1935 there were 178 operations. From 1936 to 1947 more than 1,900 persons (1,494 women and 407 men) in North Carolina were subjected to eugenic sterilization (table 6). In 1950 Moya Woodside, a sociologist who had studied the North Carolina program, concluded that it would have been even more successful had it not been for procedural difficulties, some religious opposition, the apathy of the uneducated ("especially Negroes"), indifference of the medical profession, and a shortage of surgeons. Thirty-eight county welfare officers had told her that the "red tape" of consent forms and court hearings constituted a major obstacle, and 35 other officials had identified a lack of medical facilities as a major problem.[35]

In at least a few states, the increase in the number of sterilizations is particularly striking when it is compared to the number of admissions. For example, in 1938 the Minnesota School for Feeble-Minded, in Faribault, admitted 452 patients and sterilized 151.[36] Assuming that inmates who

Table 6   Sterilizations in North Carolina, 1929-1947

		Male		Female	
Year	Total	Vasectomy	Castration	Salpingectomy	Ovariectomy
1947	122	16	3	103	—
1946	57	7	—	50	—
1945	117	15	3	98	1
1944	107	18	2	87	—
1943	152	29	4	119	—
1942	148	32	4	112	—
1941	181	45	4	132	—
1940	159	45	2	112	—
1939	138	34	2	102	—
1938	202	53	3	144	2
1937	128	18	3	105	2
1936	98	11	1	86	—
1935	178	17	7	152	2
1934	61	7	8	45	1
1933	4	1	—	3	—
1932	18	—	9	7	2
1931	11	—	—	10	1
1930	17	—	2	10	5
1929	3	1	1	—	1
	1,901	349	58	1,477	17

Note: These data are abstracted from various replies of North Carolina officials to eugenics questionnaires.

were profoundly retarded were not usually sterilized, and that many new patients were young children, it is probable that virtually every new patient in his or her reproductive years was promptly sterilized.

Throughout the 1930s California continued to have the nation's largest eugenic sterilization program (table 7). From 1923 through 1926, the annual number of sterilizations in California climbed from 190 to 541. During the next six years (1927-32) a total of 3,327 operations were performed—about 550 per year. The numbers continued to climb: in 1935 alone there were 870 sterilizations. From 1930 through 1944, nearly 11,000 persons were sterilized in California institutions.

The dramatic increase in the sterilizations performed annually is reflected by the appearance of many new programs as well as by the sharp increase in the level of activity of established ones. In 1920, twelve states had eugenic sterilization programs; by 1927, there were programs in nine-

Table 7 Sterilizations of Institutionalized Persons in California (1909-1945)

Year	Annual Total	Year	Annual Total	Year	Annual Total
1945	436	1932		1920	118
1944		1931		1919	320
1943	219	1930		1918	455
1942		1929		1917	375
1941	652	1928	532	1916	182
1940	842	1927	435	1915	116
1939	785	1926	541	1914	91
1938	761	1925	396	1913	120
1937	696	1924	316	1912	80
1936	683	1923	190	1911	148
1935	870	1922	208	1910	11
1934		1921	153	1909	0
1933					

Note: These data are abstracted from responses by California officials to various eugenics questionnaires over the years.

teen states; and in 1932, there were programs in twenty-seven states. The major change occurred in 1929. During 1927 and 1928, 2,271 sterilizations were performed in the nation's institutions, while in 1929 alone there were 2,362 operations. From 1929 through 1941, more than 2,000 eugenic sterilizations were performed each year in the United States. The most active year was 1932, when there were 3,921 reported operations.

Although there is little discussion of the Depression in the reports compiled by the various state institutions in the 1930s, during that era sterilization procedures were almost certainly being influenced by harsh economic realities. In an era when there were no funds to build more institutions, a program of paroling the less retarded in favor of admitting the more seriously retarded was one obvious solution to reduce serious overcrowding. This reinforced arguments in favor of sterilizing mildly retarded young women. Follow-up studies of such women after parole seemed to validate this policy. For example, a 1928 Wisconsin study found that half of the women discharged after being sterilized were successfully working as domestics. The study concluded: "Many mentally deficient persons by consenting to the operation are permitted to return, under supervision, to society where they become self-supporting social units and acceptable citizens. Those inmates unwilling to consent to the operation remain segregated for social protection as well as individual wel-

fare."[37] Clearly, for the many mildly retarded persons who could understand the option being presented to them, parole was a powerful incentive
to submit to the surgery.

A 1926 Minnesota study also reported that most of the persons sterilized under the new law "had been released to live in normal society."[38] In
1928 state officials followed up on a group of 147 women who had been
sterilized and found that more than 100 were no longer institutionalized.
They concluded that "sterilization is making possible many paroles which
could not otherwise have been planned for, and that most are successful."[39] The study did not address the possibility that those women had not
needed to be institutionalized. In 1934, acknowledging that "the increase
in the number of feeble-minded and epileptic persons who are yearly committed to the guardianship of the Board continues far ahead of the state's
building program for these groups," Minnesota officials again reported
that the sterilization program was permitting the release of inmates. The
parole figures are impressive. In 1921-22, when no sterilizations took
place, 70 persons were paroled. During 1931-32, 146 persons were sterilized, most of whom were among the 280 persons who were paroled.
During 1933 and 1934, at least 369 persons were paroled, of whom 213
had been sterilized.

A South Dakota study of the costs of sterilization and parole relative
to lifetime institutionalization concluded that "the average cost to maintain
patients in their own homes was less than would have been required to
maintain them in the institution."[40] A survey of sterilization in Virginia
reported that 729 of the first 1,000 persons who were sterilized had eventually been placed "in their own or suitable foster homes." It concluded
that sterilization had "proven its value."[41] A New Hampshire study of
sterilized persons who were paroled from the Laconia State School between 1928 and 1938 found that they were more likely to succeed than
nonsterilized persons who were paroled. Because their stay in the institution had on average been briefer, they had also cost the state less money
than had the nonsterilized parole group.[42]

These reports did not explain how eugenic sterilization enhanced the
chances of a successful parole. Of course, the operation eliminated the
chance that a particular feeble-minded woman might bear children, some
of whom might become wards of the state. Feeble-minded men who were
discharged after being sterilized were also protected from the burdens of
parenthood, but the likelihood of a retarded man becoming a parent was
probably substantially less than the chance of a retarded woman becoming
pregnant.

Sterilization Abroad

Eugenic victories in the United States were replicated in other nations. During the 1920s and 1930s, laws to prevent procreation by the feeble-minded and/or insane were enacted in Canada, Denmark, Germany, Sweden, Norway, Finland, Mexico, Japan, and France. England was the only major nation in which the proponents of sterilization were unequivocally rejected. Swiss physicians were probably the first to perform eugenic sterilizations. The most influential advocate was Auguste Henri Forel, a famous neurologist who directed a psychiatric clinic at the University of Zurich. From its start in the late 1890s, his sterilization program was considered part of the therapeutic arsenal to help mentally ill patients. Such operations, however, were only performed electively after obtaining consent from the patient and his or her family.[43] Unfortunately, the thorough, deliberative manner in which the Swiss psychiatrists invoked the sterilization option was not followed elsewhere.

Given the influence of Galton, it is hardly surprising that proposals favoring eugenic sterilization arose early in England. Even before Galton and his followers organized the Eugenics Education Society (EES) in 1907, other writers were championing sterilization. The most outspoken was Robert Reid Rentoul, a Liverpool physician who in 1903 published a book entitled *Proposed Sterilization of Certain Mental and Physical Degenerates.* This inflammatory tract earned him considerable notoriety, but his extremist views probably harmed the nascent eugenics movement. In 1909 another Englishman, Carl Saleeby, published *Parenthood and Race Culture*, a somewhat less radical work that made a better case for sterilization, giving it a relatively modest place in a program of positive eugenics.

In its early years the EES was quite successful. As one historian put it, "Almost the entire biological establishment joined the Eugenics Education Society and many of the most distinguished geneticists took an active part in its day to day work." By 1914 many cities had chapters, and the EES counted six hundred dues-paying members. Part of the reason for its success was that the EES espoused moderate views. Although they favored voluntary sterilization, officials in London and at the important Cambridge chapter rejected calls for compulsory sterilization as premature. As the secretary of the Cambridge chapter put it, "We are more or less in the dark as to the physical, mental and moral effects of [sterilization], not to mention the serious ethical problems that are raised."[44]

In 1904 there was sufficient controversy over how best to care for mental defectives that a Royal Commission was formed to study the matter.

When it issued its report four years later, the commission concluded that there were large numbers of mentally defective persons whose care had been seriously neglected. Major recommendations from this study were embodied in the Mental Deficiency Act of 1913, which greatly encouraged the development of training programs and housing for the handicapped, and which rejected proposals for eugenic sterilization.[45]

A little more than a decade later, partly in response to the rapidly escalating financial needs of the state hospitals, the EES decided to propose voluntary sterilization for the mentally deficient. In 1928 it published a pamphlet that included the draft of a sterilization bill. By 1931 there was sufficient support for the idea that the bill was introduced in the House of Commons. The Commons rejected the proposal but directed the minister of health to appoint a special committee to explore the matter. The unanimous conclusion of the Brock Committee (named for its chairman) was to reject compulsory sterilization but to approve cautiously the selective use of voluntary sterilization.[46]

The Brock Report was influenced by two 1933 studies, one by the Mental Deficiency Committee of the British Medical Association and the other by Dr. Alfred Turner, which rejected key arguments of the pro-sterilization forces. As for the contention that most mentally defective persons had inherited their affliction, the British Medical Association stated flatly that the pedigree studies (largely compiled by the Eugenics Record Office at Cold Spring Harbor) upon which this assertion was based were flawed and that it was "not proved that feeble-mindedness is inherited on Mendelian lines."[47] Later that year Dr. Alfred Turner, a prominent British physician, sharply attacked the idea that defective persons had unusually large families. His study of the graduates of the Birmingham Special Schools showed just the opposite result. Contrary to the findings of the ERO's pedigree studies, Turner's study also demonstrated that only 5 percent of feeble-minded persons had feeble-minded parents or grandparents. He concluded: "The statement if all mental defectives could be prevented from having children, the number of defectives would be halved in three generations is not only untrue, but one for which there is no foundation in any knowledge we at present possess."[48] Despite intermittent lobbying efforts by eugenicists over the next three decades, Great Britain never adopted a program of eugenic sterilization.

Perhaps because of their proximity to the United States, two of the Canadian provinces broke with England and adopted sterilization laws. The first and more important was Alberta, which implemented a program in 1928. Defining a retardate as "someone having an arrested or incomplete development of mind existing before 18 years of age," the law empowered a four-person eugenics board to consider petitions to sterilize such persons. Over a forty-three-year period, 2,822 persons were sterilized under Alberta's law. Given the province's relatively small population, this was one of the world's more robust programs. In its final year (1971), the Eugenics Board considered seventy-eight petitions and approved seventy-seven; fifty-five persons were sterilized.[49]

In addition to Great Britain and the United States, Germany was the other nation in which eugenic ideas took root at the turn of the century. Although it is possible to trace the movement well into the nineteenth century, real interest in eugenics in Germany began about 1890. In his last writings, the immensely popular philosopher Friedrich Nietzsche urged a variety of eugenic measures, including segregation, to protect the Nordic race. In 1895 Otto Seeck published *The Downfall of the Ancient World,* in which he argued that Greek civilization had fallen largely owing to dysgenic influences, and that the German people were similarly threatened. That year Alfred Ploetz, a physician who had been trained in the United States, published a book, *Foundations of a Eugenics,* in which he made a strong pro-sterilization plea. Another book for laymen, *Heredity and Selection in the Life of Peoples,* which appeared in 1903, won a eugenics contest sponsored by the Krupp steel family.[50]

In 1904 Ploetz, the Galton of German eugenics, founded the first journal devoted to the study of race hygiene, and in 1905 he organized the German Eugenics Society. In 1907, thanks in part to the society's efforts, a sterilization bill was discussed in the Reichstag, but it was rejected. At the International Hygiene Exposition held in Dresden in 1911, the society sponsored an exhibit on eugenics. By 1914 it was sufficiently well organized to be meeting regularly and to publish a set of eugenic principles. The war years interrupted the German eugenics movement, but by the 1920s interest was again on the rise. In 1923, Bavaria became the first of the German states to create a university chair in eugenics. In that year, three of Germany's leading biologists, Ernst Bauer, Ernst Fisher, and Fritz Lenz, published a book on "race hygiene" that sold well. About the same time, German writers also began to publish books that argued the genetic superiority of the Nordic race.[51]

In October 1921, the German Society for Race Hygiene adopted a forty-one-point eugenics program. Largely focused on positive eugenics, the tract is surprising for the firm voice with which it rejected the idea of compulsory eugenic sterilization. Although it favored the right of defective individuals "to be sterilized by their own wish," it pursued a policy of segregation and urged the creation of self-supporting labor colonies rather than adopting a policy of "bodily injury." Writing about sterilization in

1924, one German eugenicist acknowledged that "in a legislative way practically nothing has yet been done among us," but he consoled himself that "too hasty legislation in this matter may also provoke disastrous reactions."[52]

About this time, Adolph Hitler, who was quite taken with eugenics notions, was writing *Mein Kampf* in a German prison. In *Mein Kampf*, Hitler wrote: "To prevent defective persons from reproducing equally defective offspring, is an act dictated by the clearest light of reason. Its carrying out is the most humane act of mankind. It would prevent the unmerited suffering of millions of persons, and, above all would, in the end, result in a steady increase in human welfare."[53] Perhaps the most striking aspect of these words is their similarity to those of Justice Oliver Wendell Holmes, who wrote the opinion in *Buck v. Bell.*

Shortly after the Nazis came to power, they enacted a comprehensive state health program, one prominent feature of which was incentives to encourage earlier marriages and larger families. A marriage loan fund helped young adults purchase homes at interest rates adjusted to their ability to pay. Municipal governments were ordered to help defray the costs of raising the third and fourth children in a family, special subsidies were offered to economically stressed farmers, and bachelors and childless couples were made to pay more income tax than did parents of several children.[54]

A comprehensive German eugenic sterilization law was enacted on July 14, 1933, and went into effect on January 1, 1934. In the summer of 1936 Marie Kopp, who worked for the American Committee on Maternal Health, set out to conduct a detailed study of the origin, operation, and impact of the German law. She spent several months observing and interviewing many judges of the "Hereditary Health Courts." One of the things she discovered was that the German translation of *Sterilization for Human Betterment,* by Gosney and Popenoe, had been extremely influential: "The leaders in the sterilization movement in Germany tell one over and over again that their sterilization legislation was formulated after careful study of the California experiment under Mr. Gosney and Dr. Popenoe's leadership."[55]

The influence of the American eugenicists can be found in other nations as well. For example, in 1927 Laughlin wrote to Judge Harry Olson to urge that a copy of his sterilization book be sent to Dr. H. O. Wildenskon in Brejning, Denmark. At the time Wildenskon, an assistant medical director of the state institution for mental defectives, was a member of a special commission to investigate the use of eugenic sterilization. In 1928 Denmark did enact a sterilization law.[56]

The German eugenicists were especially impressed with Laughlin's work on eugenic sterilization. About 1921 Laughlin, an acknowledged Germanophile, began to write articles about the eugenics movement in Germany for *Eugenics News.* During the late 1920s and early 1930s, he also wrote several articles on sterilization for German journals. In 1936, at the height of Germany's sterilization campaign, Laughlin and several other Americans were awarded honorary doctoral degrees by Heidelberg University.[57]

The German sterilization law empowered special courts to approve the sterilization of persons about whom, in "the experience of medical science, it may be expected with great probability that their offspring may suffer severe physical damage." Whether motivated by considerations of due process or by a concern for efficiency, the law also warned that surgeons who sterilized patients without appropriate authorization from public health officials were subject to malpractice litigation and criminal prosecution. It fell to public health officials to identify persons who were likely to bear defective children, but who were unlikely or unwilling to undergo "voluntary" sterilization. Generally such persons were brought to the attention of local officials by superintendents of institutions for the retarded, physicians, or next of kin. If the local public health worker felt that an individual should be sterilized, that official petitioned the Hereditary Health Court to consider the case. At first there were nine conditions for which sterilization was compulsory: inborn feeble-mindedness, schizophrenia, manic-depressive insanity, hereditary epilepsy, Huntington's chorea, hereditary blindness, hereditary deafness, severe hereditary physical deformity, and severe habitual drunkenness.[58]

Each Hereditary Health Court had three members; a district judge presided, and a public health officer and a physician assisted with the eugenic determination. The sterilization hearings were largely decided on the basis of the medical reports. Some courts did not even call the individual to the hearing. Either party (public health authority or patient) had the right to appeal the court's finding to a special court of appeals, but its ruling was final.

In implementing the law, German officials took two measures to reduce opposition: they forbade the sterilization of children who had not entered the reproductive years, and they ruled that no Roman Catholic judge or surgeon could be forced to participate in a sterilization case. Further, they agreed not to sterilize a Catholic patient who remained in an institution at the expense of his family or the church.[59]

The scale of the German sterilization program during the mid-1930s dwarfed all prior programs. In 1934 alone, 205 Hereditary Health Courts received 84,525 applications for sterilization. Of these, 64,499 (73 percent) were heard and decided. Sterilization was ordered in 56,244 cases (28,286 men and 27,958 women), for a "eugenic conviction rate" of 87 percent. The higher courts heard 8,219 appeals, of which half were successful. Thus, about 52,000 persons were placed under final order to be sterilized in Germany during the program's first year. During 1935 the courts continued to consider sterilization petitions at a rapid pace. By July 1, after only eighteen months of operation, about 150,000 persons had been ordered sterilized. Roughly speaking, each of the lower courts decided about 3 cases a day, a level of judicial efficiency that almost certainly indicates that only the most superficial review of sterilization petitions was ever made.[60]

The German sterilization law had an obvious impact on the medical literature pertaining to sterilization. Review of the *Quarterly Cumulative Index to Current Medical Literature* from 1921 through 1932 indicates that about 20 articles appeared annually. In 1933, the year of the new German law, the number of articles (most of them written in German) jumped from 26 to 42. The following year there were 94 articles, followed by 96 in 1935 and 75 in 1936. After 1936 the number of publications fell off. The German literature fell into two categories: articles concerned with the organization of the program and the psychological and physical sequelae of sterilization on the patients, and articles that presented new evidence for a genetic component of various handicaps, thus extending the size of the population that fell under the jurisdiction of the Hereditary Health Courts. By the late 1930s, eugenic ideology even seemed to be influencing the conduct of medical research. For example, a Canadian physician published a paper titled "Leber's Hereditary Optic Neuritis through Six Generations: A Sterilization Problem."[61]

In the United States, eugenicists hailed the German program and characterized it as a sensible plan that was working well. One writer, describing the manner in which the Hereditary Health Courts dealt with "borderline cases," concluded that their rulings were "conservative." He noted one court's refusal to sterilize a farmer with tuberculosis and another's refusal to sterilize a music student of exceptional talent whose family had a history of manic-depressive illness.[62] In the same year, however, Fritz Lenz, the leading scientific eugenicist in Germany, proposed to sterilize all carriers of defective genes—a group then thought to include one-fifth of the population.[63]

During the middle and late 1930s, the German sterilization program cast an ever larger net. Late in 1934 the German Supreme Court ruled that the sterilization law applied to non-Germans living in Germany. During

1935 and 1936, there was an avalanche of petitions and articles praising the economic advantages of the program. Other nations listened; in 1934 Norway and Sweden adopted sterilization laws, followed the next year by Finland. All were roughly modeled on the German approach. The 1934 Swedish law authorized the sterilization of persons lacking legal capacity who were likely to bear children with a hereditary defect or "were unable to assume the legal and moral responsibility for proper fostering of children." Although it permitted the family or guardian of a person to speak at the hearing, the law did not require their consent for surgery.[64]

During the period 1935-39, Sweden operated a relatively vigorous sterilization program. In four years its medical board ordered 350 involuntary sterilizations. By an alternative legal route another 472 persons, all of whom were feeble-minded, were sterilized each after two physicians had concluded that it would be beneficial. There were 2,093 sterilizations performed in Sweden during this period (822 were compulsory, and 1,271 by the "patient's request"). The vast majority (1,912) were women, of whom 13 died during the surgery. Well after World War II (1948-49), this lightly populated nation was sterilizing over 2,000 persons each year, a cohort in which about half the operations were involuntary.[65]

Because so many records were destroyed during World War II we will never know how many persons were sterilized under the German law. In 1951, the Central Association of Sterilized People in West Germany charged that from 1933 to 1945, the Nazis sterilized 3,500,000 people. Since this is nearly double the number of hereditary defectives assumed by even the most paranoid German eugenicists to live on German soil, it suggests that the program quickly lost all restraint. For example, the chairman of the Central Association, Bruno Koeniger, claimed that he was sterilized late in 1933 for the sole reason that he was half-Jewish. He recalled that "a nervous breakdown, a suicide attempt, a vague suspicion was sufficient evidence for the Nazis to wipe out an undesirable." Koeniger also asserted that as the years passed the Nazis sterilized an even larger percentage of women.[66]

The German documents that survived World War II do suggest that by 1940-41 the sterilization program had veered far from its original course. Consider a memo signed by Oberführer Gregor Elsner, an obstetrician who decided the fate of many Rumanian children kidnapped for the Lebensborn program. On August 25, 1941, commenting on the reproductive fitness of these children, Elsner wrote, "Also two of the boys should immediately be made incapable of reproduction, one of them, Nikolaus Reiszer, because he has tuberculosis and the other, George Kuhn, because with his protruding ears and round shoulders he makes an impression of degeneracy."[67]

By 1940, as they plunged into World War II, German authorities chose ever more grim methods to accomplish their goals. During the Nuremberg trials, evidence was presented by SHAEF intelligence that between June 1940 and July 1941 there were many executions of patients suffering from "severe" mental defect or illness. According to a secret file that survived orders that it be destroyed, 1,857 retarded German patients were taken from the Munich area to be killed in Poland. It was reported that in Egfling several hundred retarded children were killed with poison by a squad of "nurses" sent from Berlin. The file includes copies of letters of inquiry sent by relatives and examples of the various lies (death by appendicitis) concocted to cover up the mass murders. Apparently, enough German people were outraged that the practice of killing fellow Germans, however retarded, was halted in late 1942.[68]

The German sterilization program, from its inception in 1934 until it ended in 1945, far eclipsed similar American activities. Eugenic sterilization in Germany was not veiled in secrecy. To the contrary, it was openly reported, and it provided a model for other European countries. There is, thus, little foundation for the not uncommon assertion that postwar revulsion over Nazi crimes helped to end American sterilization programs. Indeed, a number of states maintained busy programs in the 1940s and 1950s.

8 · Critics

Our statistics definitely indicate that there is no real increase in the commitment rate and that biologically, so far as mental disease is concerned the race is not rapidly going to the dogs, as has been the favorite assertion for some time.

—Abraham Myerson, Committee of the American Neurological
Association for the Investigation of Eugenical Sterilization, 1935

It is no surprise that psychometrics should have had its share of bigots. What is regrettable is that they have so often lent the mantle of their science to prejudice, leaving to outsiders the job of exposing errors.

—Nicholas Wade, *New York Times*, September 11, 1982

The difficulty in understanding why hereditarian notions once held such appeal for the American mind is matched by the challenge of explaining how more enlightened thinking supplanted them. But in poking through dusty, long-unread journals and the archives of men not quite important enough to deserve library space, one does find a few hints. At different times leading geneticists, social scientists, physicians, and, especially, the Catholic church attacked sterilization programs. More recently, civil libertarians, lawyers, and patients' families sharply rejected the old notions.

Geneticists

The central dogma of the eugenics movement was that virtually all human defects could be ultimately explained by the presence of one or more genetically determined characteristics. In the first decade of this century, Charles Davenport led the drive to redefine humankind in Mendelian terms. Pedigree studies of single gene disorders like Huntington disease provided convincing evidence of the wisdom of this enterprise. But eugenicists failed to maintain the discipline and doubt of their colleagues who studied fruit flies, corn, and mice. With little scientific support, Davenport and his followers baldly asserted that most persons who suffered from feeble-mindedness, epilepsy, and insanity were cursed with one or more of a variety of deleterious genes that had sealed their fate at conception. Using crude and uncontrolled methods to gather data, eugenicists (who thought of themselves as human geneticists) also claimed that criminality, prostitution, and pauperism were largely due to genetically controlled encephalopathies. Davenport went so far as to declare that men who ran off to sea did so under the influence of a sex-linked gene, a condition he dubbed "thalassophilia."[1]

During the heyday of eugenics the science of genetics was making extraordinary strides. At Columbia University, Thomas Hunt Morgan led some brilliant graduate students in the painstaking analysis of the chromosomes of the fruit fly, *Drosophila melanogaster.* Leaving the "fly room," these younger men started their own laboratories in other universities and charted a course that their intellectual grandchildren steer today. Their work was slow and careful; it often required months of study and the examination of thousands of flies to map a unit character to a particular chromosome. Given their rigorous standards, it is likely that not a few of them were critical of Laughlin, Estabrook, and their ilk. Surely, as they saw immigration restriction and involuntary sterilization programs justified with eugenic evidence, they must have questioned the validity of those data. In the 1920s a few leading geneticists were openly critical of eugenics, but most kept silent.

The silence is not difficult to explain. During the first four decades of this century there were only a few hundred geneticists in the United States. Scattered across the nation's universities, they spent their days at the laboratory benches, nurturing their flies with mashed bananas and meticulously counting thousands of offspring from planned matings. Even if they had wished to join the political fray, their jobs demanded too much of their time and, doubtless, the manner in which they studied heredity had little impact in the corridors of power. As one historian has written: "Because balanced geneticists rarely wrote on man, the new developments remained largely hidden from the educated public, and eugenists continued their domination of human genetics."[2]

Another reason why relatively few geneticists spoke out against eugenic sterilization programs was that they lacked a formal method for disproving the theories that had fostered these programs' implementation. With the exception of the Hardy-Weinberg law, which demonstrated that variability is preserved in a randomly breeding population, the foundations of population genetics were not developed until the 1920s and 1930s. Given this fact, it is interesting that shortly after it was proven (about 1915) that selection was ineffective when targeted against an uncommon recessive gene, R. C. Punnett, a leading geneticist, used this finding to refute the eugenicists' claim that sterilization would eliminate recessively determined feeble-mindedness in a few generations.[3]

As genetics matured, the simplistic hereditarian notions embraced by eugenicists became less tenable. The discovery by Muller in 1927 that radiation could be used to create mutations in experimental organisms was an important event in the decline of eugenics. Certainly, it made the retrospective family studies so favored by the Eugenics Record Office seem woefully unscientific. During the 1930s, eugenics ceased to be regarded as a science, and most real geneticists apparently did not take it seriously enough to oppose it. Nevertheless, they did not officially condemn eugenics until after World War II, by which time other forces had already caused its demise.[4]

During the 1920s and 1930s a few prominent geneticists did speak out against eugenics. Dr. Herbert Jennings, a prominent protozoan zoologist at the Johns Hopkins Hospital, offered a sharp critique of the "Analysis of America's Modern Melting Pot," the report presented by Laughlin to Congress in support of the 1924 immigration bill. Jennings's most widely read critique, "Undesirable Aliens," appeared in the *Survey,* a popular magazine, on December 15, 1923. He argued that Laughlin's "impression that Europe falls into two contrasted regions, one desirable, the other undesirable—the north and west on the one hand, the south and east on the other" was erroneous.[5] A few months later he published a caustic review of the same material in *Science,* arguing that there was "no basis" for Laughlin's assertion that a percentage limitation based on the census of 1890 would reduce the flow of defective germ plasm.[6] His comments appeared too late to influence immigration policy.

Yet, as late as 1930 even Jennings regarded feeble-mindedness as "doubtless the clearest case" of a defect caused by a single gene pair—the view regularly advanced by eugenicists to support sterilization programs. This dramatically illustrates the extent to which a simplistic Mendelism controlled hereditarian thought in those years. Jennings opposed sterilizing the feeble minded largely because he believed that the insignificant improvement it would provide to the gene pool was outweighed by the dangerous political precedent that it constituted. He did, however, acknowledge that a sterilization program based on accurate diagnostic methods would be scientifically defensible.[7]

As did Jennings, the other geneticists who spoke forcefully against eugenics devoted significantly more energy to the immigration question than to the wisdom of sterilizing the feeble-minded. There were some volleys fired, however, at the pedigree studies that had rationalized eugenic sterilization. For example T. H. Morgan, then the dean of American genetics, pointed out that people like the Jukes and Kallikaks "lived under demoralizing social conditions that might swamp a family of average persons."[8] But Morgan, a scientists' scientist, generally shunned the political arena.

Raymond Pearl, director of the Institute for Biological Research at the Johns Hopkins University, was a strident critic of eugenics, a zeal that may have been fueled partly by memories of earlier years when he had embraced its cause. In the autumn of 1927 Pearl wrote a devastating critique of the pedigree studies that had been regularly conducted by eugenicists since Galton's work in the 1860s. He warned: "In preaching as they do, that like produces like, and that superior people will have superior children and inferior people inferior children, the orthodox eugenicists are going contrary to the best established facts of genetical science, and are, in the long run, doing their cause harm." He urged eugenics to clean its house and to throw away "the old-fashioned rubbish which has accumulated in the attic."[9]

The Nazis' dismissal of thousands of scholars from their posts in 1933 and the excesses of the German sterilization program probably stimulated some American geneticists to cast a critical eye on American eugenics.[10] But Muller was one of very few scientists who made clear their abhorrence of the racist attitudes that permeated eugenic thought. Asked to speak at the Third International Congress of Eugenics in 1932, he prepared a critique of the scientific weakness of eugenic claims. When Davenport, the program chairman, read a preprint of his paper, "The Dominance of Economics over Eugenics," he was sufficiently upset to slash Muller's podium time from one hour to ten minutes. Despite this, Muller still delivered a heavy volley against his staunchly eugenic listeners. Arguing that there was "no hard and fast line between the fit and the unfit," he asserted that fitness itself was far more than the product of a few specified genes. He urged the audience to admit that the biological forces that shaped the human condition were far beyond their understanding. Muller, an avowed socialist who was for a time enamored of communism, believed that advances in human evolution depended far more on a "socially directed economic system" than on genes.[11]

As late as 1943 E. A. Hooton, a Harvard anthropologist and avowed eugenicist, criticized "the apathy of geneticists toward the human applications of their science." Hooton accused them of a "pusillánimous and escapist attitude" and urged them to "emerge from their refuges among insects and the lower vertebrates and tackle their own species." His words confirm that few geneticists openly repudiated eugenics.[12]

Social Scientists

Some of the most articulate critics of eugenics in general and sterilization in particular came from the social sciences. At the turn of the century Social Darwinism was still hotly debated, and there was much discussion as to whether social programs should be developed to help the downtrodden and underprivileged. The pervasive but unproven belief in the high fecundity of the poor was a crucial element in that debate. Even some otherwise liberal academics such as Dartmouth sociologist Colin Wells argued that the poor were weakening society. But most agreed with Harvard's Lester Ward, the dean of the field and a critic of eugenics. He replied sharply that

> the doctrine defended by Professor Wells is the most complete example of the oligocentric world-view which is coming to prevail in the higher classes of society, and would center the entire attention of the world upon an almost infinitesimal fraction of the human race and ignore all the rest. . . .
>
> For an indefinite period yet to come society will continue to be recruited, as Mr. Benjamin Kidd well says, from the base. The swarming and spawning millions of the lower ranks will continue in the future as in the past to swamp all the fruits of intelligence and compel society to assimilate this mass of crude material as best it can. This is commonly looked upon as the deplorable consequence of the demographic law referred to, and it is said that society is doomed to hopeless degeneracy.
>
> Is it possible to take any other view? I think it is, and the only consolation, the only hope, lies in the truth—I call it a truth without hesitation, although, so far as I am aware, I am the only one to emphasize it, and perhaps the only one to accept it—that, so far as the native capacity, the potential quality, the "promise and potency," of a higher life are concerned, those swarming, spawning millions, the bottom layer of society, the proletariat, the working classes, the "hewers of wood and drawers of water," nay, even the denizens of the slums—that all these are by nature the peers of the boasted "aristocracy of brains" that now dominates society and looks down upon them, and the equals in all but privilege of the most enlightened teachers of eugenics.[13]

In academic circles, at least, the most important critic of eugenics was German-born Franz Boas, the father of anthropology in the United States.

During his long tenure at Columbia University Boas trained Ruth Benedict, Margaret Mead, Alfred Kroeber, Robert Lowe, and Ruth Burzel, men and women who shaped the field of cultural anthropology. Originally trained in physics, in the early 1880s he became fascinated with ethnology and spent a year among the Eskimo near Baffin Island. Returning to Berlin, he studied with Rudolph Virchow, the leading German anthropologist, who was deeply opposed to Darwin's theory of evolution. Another influence was Theodore Waitz, who in 1859 had published a work that strongly embraced cultural determinism. Virchow's antievolutionism and Waitz's strongly argued view that environment far exceeded the shaping force of natural endowment led Boas to give little value to the nature side of the great nature/nurture debate of which the eugenics movement was a manifestation.[14] Beginning in the mid-1890s, Boas's major intellectual goal was "to distinguish the concepts of race and culture, to separate biological and cultural heredity, to focus attention on cultural process, to free the concept of culture from its heritage of evolutionary and racial assumption, so that it could subsequently become . . . completely independent of biological determinism."[15] His first major attack on eugenics resulted from an invitation from Congress to study the assimilability of young immigrants. From his detailed anthropomorphic and cultural assessment of young Sicilian and Hebrew immigrants on the lower east side of Manhattan in 1909 he concluded that once they learned the English language and American ways, the newcomers would flourish.[16] He thus discredited ideas that had been advanced by the Immigration Restriction League and others who believed that the newcomers threatened the nation's racial vigor.

While he stood virtually alone in his outspoken criticism of eugenics from about 1905 to 1920, after that point Boas was joined by other colleagues in cultural anthropology and related disciplines. One strategy employed by the critics was to use field studies to test theories of biological determinism. The most famous example is undoubtedly Margaret Mead's study of female adolescence in the South Seas. Her book *Coming of Age in Samoa* portrayed a society in which adolescence was the easiest, calmest period in the life cycle, free from the storms that characterized American teenage life, which many people thought were predetermined.[17]

While Boas and his students, joined by J. B. Watson and his students in the new field of behavioral psychology, posed a counterweight to eugenic thinking, few scientists, if any, singled out involuntary sterilization for criticism. The anthropologists devoted their energies to the larger question of the extent to which racial differences were genetically or culturally influenced. The social scientists who criticized eugenics and offered the intellectual alternative of cultural determinism certainly helped to end its dominance, but they had no obvious impact on sterilization programs.

About 1940 some sociologists did begin to investigate sterilization. One professor at the University of Detroit wrote to the Carnegie Institute asking:

> Can you tell me why counsel for Carrie Buck did not oppose her sterilization, at the several stages of her case through the courts, on the grounds that none of the three generations were proven to suffer from "mental defect," not to say "hereditary"? Could you kindly say, too, what Carrie Buck's subsequent history has been? Also, and more particularly, in the thirteen years since the disposal of this case, has Carrie Buck's child proven to be a mental defective, and this despite reasonably good developmental opportunities?[18]

These were good questions. In fact, neither Carrie Buck nor her daughter were mentally retarded. It was not until the 1940s that the thesis that most retarded persons were born to retarded persons (the key tenet of sterilization programs) was flatly rejected. In his influential book, *The Biology of Mental Defect*, Lionel Penrose, a leading British scientist, wrote, "Owing to the fact that the great majority of defectives of all grades are born to parents who cannot be classed as defective themselves, the reduction of defect in the community by preventing all known cases from having children would not be spectacular."[19] As for sterilization of criminals and other socially inadequate persons, Penrose asserted that the idea that social inefficiency "can be prevented on the basis of genetical theory is essentially invalid."[20]

With the late 1940s came a new concern for the retarded, largely fueled by their own families. In 1950 the National Association of Parents and Friends of Mentally Deficient Children was formed. Renamed the National Association for Retarded Children (NARC), this vigorous organization soon had chapters in every state, and within a decade it matured into a powerful lobby.

Within the mental health community, the transition in attitude from the dark days of the 1930s to the brighter outlook of the 1950s was not untroubled. Admitting that the original hereditarian thesis had been overstated, sterilization advocates dressed their arguments in a new costume, stressing the benefits conferred by the operation. As one psychologist wrote, "On medical and humanitarian grounds we are being unjust in not discouraging mentally defective individuals from bearing offspring."[21] The rhetoric of the "menace" of the feeble-minded had quieted, but the policy goals of an earlier day lingered.

The Catholic Church

Given the church's longstanding position on birth control, it is hardly surprising to learn that Catholic theologians were among the earliest critics of eugenic sterilization in the United States. When the laws were first enacted (1907-15), theologians asked whether the sterilization of retarded persons, the insane, or criminals could find moral justification within Catholic doctrine. Although the majority opposed the sterilization operation because it destroyed a "natural faculty," a minority view emerged that sought to accommodate sterilization. For example Samuel Donovan, of St. Bonaventure's Seminary in New York, argued that if the public welfare was sufficiently threatened by large numbers of degenerate persons, it would be morally permissible to sterilize them. He premised his argument in part on the fact that Catholic doctrine accepted capital punishment as necessary to preserve order in society. Several other Catholic scholars seconded this position.[22]

Theological discussion of the sterilization problem subsided in intensity during World War I, but with the second wave of sterilization laws in the twenties, the level of moral discourse grew. This was in part because the proponents of eugenic sterilization also wished to stem the tide of immigrants. This directly threatened the Catholic church, a church of immigrants.

By the mid-1920s, representatives of Catholic dioceses and lay Catholic groups were often the most important opponents of eugenic sterilization proposals. In 1927 the governor of Colorado vetoed a sterilization bill, in part owing to opposition from the Holy Name Society and the Denver Knights of Columbus. The Denver Diocesan Holy Name Union condemned the bill both because it violated natural law and because it posed a high risk of flagrant injustice owing to "human inability to pass judgment on human mentality." Roswell Johnson, who monitored legislative developments for *Eugenics* magazine, reported that Roman Catholics had also "furnished the main opposition to the New York and Connecticut birth control bills."[23] Also in 1927 John A. Ryan, a professor of theology at Catholic University and a spokesman for the Vatican on policy issues in the United States, broke ranks with his more reform-minded colleagues on the National Catholic Welfare Council to condemn eugenic sterilization as a violation of the "intrinsic sacredness of the person." However, even he did not exclude the possibility that under certain conditions the public welfare might require involuntary sterilization.[24]

In Europe (especially in Germany), during the late 1920s, a handful of Catholic scholars argued forcefully that eugenic sterilization could be morally justified. Fritz Tillman, a moral philosopher at Bonn, asserted that persons at risk for bearing defective children had an obligation to refrain from marriage and parenthood. Joseph Mayer, who crusaded in favor of eugenic sterilization, sought authority in the work of Thomas Aquinas, who had recognized the power of the state to castrate certain convicted criminals. Mayer's book, *The Sterilization of the Mentally Diseased,* gained much attention from Catholic scholars.[25]

In January 1930 Pope Pius XI issued *Casti Connubi (On Christian Marriage),* the first encyclical to address eugenics. *Casti Connubi* acknowledged that the aims of eugenics were good so long as "lawful and upright methods are employed within the proper limits," but it warned that "evil is not to be done that good may come of it." As for sterilization, *Casti Connubi* held:

> Finally, that pernicious practice must be condemned which closely touches upon the natural right of man to enter matrimony but affects also in a real way the welfare of the offspring. For there are some who, oversolicitous for the cause of eugenics, not only give salutary counsel for more certainly procuring the strength and health of the future child—which, indeed, is not contrary to right reason—but put eugenics before aims of a higher order, and by public authority wish to prevent from marrying all those whom, even though naturally fit for marriage, they consider, according to the norms and conjectures of their investigations, would, through hereditary transmission, bring forth defective offspring.
>
> And more, they wish to legislate to deprive these of that natural faculty by medical action despite their unwillingness, and this they do not propose as an infliction of grave punishment under the authority of the State for a crime committed, nor to prevent future crimes by guilty persons, but against every right and good they wish the civil authority to arrogate to itself a power over a faculty which it never had and can never legitimately possess.
>
> Those who act in this way are at fault in losing sight of the fact that the family is more sacred than the State and that men are begotten not for the earth and for time but for Heaven and eternity. Although often these individuals are to be dissuaded from entering into matrimony, certainly it is wrong to brand men with the stigma of crime because they contract marriage, on the ground that, despite the fact that they are in every respect capable of matrimony, they will give birth only to defective children, even though they use all care and diligence.
>
> Public magistrates have no direct power over the bodies of their subjects; therefore, where no crime has taken place and there is no cause present for grave punishment, they can never directly harm, or tamper with the integrity of the body, either for the reasons of eugenics or for any other reason. St.

Thomas teaches this when inquiring whether human judges for the sake of preventing future evils can inflict punishment, he admits that the power indeed exists as regards certain other forms of evil, but justly and properly denies it as regards the maiming of the body. No one who is guiltless may be punished by a human tribunal either by flogging to death, or mutilation, or by beating.[26]

After *Casti Connubi* Catholic lay organizations rallied to oppose sterilization bills. The Knights of Columbus and other groups responded to homilies by Catholic bishops and brought their opposition to the desks of their legislative representatives. In addition, the encyclical quieted those liberal Catholic theologians who had before its issuance adopted contrary points of view. *Casti Connubi* also thoroughly condemned elective sterilization and contraception to limit family size. In so doing, it polarized many Protestant theologians who approved of birth control and may have driven a few of them to embrace some of the more extreme tenets of eugenics. Certainly, the clash between Protestants and Catholics over birth control had its bitter moments from the 1930s forward. By the 1940s, the Catholic church had embarked on a sustained drive against eugenic sterilization laws. For example, in 1943 the National Catholic Welfare Conference widely distributed a lengthy pamphlet written by the Reverend Edgar Schmiedeleer that condemned sterilization as a morally unacceptable means of human betterment.[27]

By 1945 Marion B. Olden, the executive secretary of Birthright (and a rabid anti-Catholic) was sure that Roman Catholic opposition constituted the "greatest obstacle" to the sterilization movement. She claimed that Quebec's Catholics had stirred up the faithful in Maine and had slowed the implementation of that state's program. She also reported that Arizona officials had told her their law was inoperable "due to religious opposition." A 1940 report to her from Wisconsin was especially detailed. The Wisconsin Race Conservation Committee had submitted a bill to enlarge the reach of the state's sterilization program. According to Olden it was defeated by the following tactics:

A priest called upon an assemblyman and told him that he controlled 1,200 votes in his parish, that these votes would be necessary for his re-election and that only by voting against the sterilization bill could he hope to be returned to the Assembly. Another assembly man was threatened with a boycott of his store by all Catholics in his district if he continued to favor the bill. Another assemblyman who was in the insurance business was told that the policies he had written on a Catholic church would not be renewed if he voted for the bill. A fourth assemblyman who published a newspaper was told that his Catholic subscribers would drop the paper.[28]

Olden also described how in 1945 a determined band of Catholics defeated a sterilization bill in Alabama, a state in which the vast majority was Protestant.

Whenever sterilization bills are introduced the Catholics descend upon the capitol in numbers—priests, nuns and laity—and attack the bill as "against the will of God" and "an attack on the American home." In 1945 they tried delaying tactics. After legislative committee hearings were called and delegations in support of the bill traveled to Montgomery, on some excuse the hearing would be postponed. A Catholic physician testified at the hearing that States with a law, including California, have ceased to use it and that the operation robs a man of virility!

The tactics used in Wisconsin were not wanting in Alabama. A legislator who was known to be a convinced proponent of sterilization had introduced a bill for cancer research funds, and was threatened by a Catholic legislator with defeat for that bill unless the sterilization bill was defeated. The bishop sent an ugly letter resigning from the State cancer control board and threatening the cancer bill. In this instance the legislator refused to be intimidated. Priests all over Alabama preached sermons against the sterilization bill, using as a main argument that it was an opening wedge in a Hitlerian program of mutilation.

Supporters of the bill brought large delegations to the hearings, including Protestant ministers, professors of biology and psychiatrists. The Federation of Women's Clubs and the American Association of University Women backed the bill. Finally after a three-day Catholic filibuster, it safely passed the Senate. In the House the sponsor jettisoned the bill in a political bargain, an event which made at least one representative decide to withdraw from politics and refuse to run in the following primaries.[29]

Olden also claimed that despite a favorable review by the State Bar Association and the support of welfare groups, Catholics in Wyoming, led by the bishop of Cheyenne, had easily defeated a proposed sterilization bill. Also in 1945 the cardinal's office in Philadelphia was instrumental in defeating a eugenic sterilization bill prepared by the Pennsylvania Psychiatric Society. The cardinal allegedly wrote to every legislator asking them to oppose the bill; priests called on the lawmakers to reiterate the message, and then they preached against the bill from the pulpits. Owing to her profound anti-Catholicism, it is possible that Olden exaggerated, but her reports leave little doubt that the Catholic church did more to repudiate eugenic sterilization than did geneticists.

Physicians

In the early days, physicians rarely emerged as critics of eugenic sterilization. Those who believed that the threat of pregnancy was a moral deterrent did worry that sterilization would increase licentiousness and foster the spread of venereal disease. As the Victorian era subsided, however, this concern claimed few adherents. During the late 1920s, physicians who opposed eugenic sterilization mainly argued that there was insufficient knowledge of human heredity to justify such measures. For example, speaking before his state medical society, a New Orleans physician argued that it was "quite impossible to predict with precision the type of offspring of any given mating."[30] But the majority seemed enthralled with Mendelism, so his was a minority view.

Perhaps the first important *medical* critique of eugenic ideas was published by Dr. Walter Fernald in 1919. For twenty-five years, Fernald, an expert in the causes of mental retardation who worked in Massachusetts, followed the lives of 646 nonsterilized feeble-minded persons after discharge from a state school. Contrary to the common belief, he found that they had a low marriage rate and a very low birth rate. Of the 176 women, only 27 had married, and they had given birth to only 50 children, of whom 33 had survived. Eleven unmarried women had borne 13 children. Of the 470 males, only 13 had married, and they had fathered only 12 children. Dr. Fernald concluded that the eugenicists had mistaken a high birth rate among poor, uneducated people for the fertility of the feeble-minded. His study seriously threatened the celebrated pedigree studies of Dugdale, Davenport, and Goddard that had provided the intellectual rationale for the eugenics movement. However, it had no immediate influence on sterilization programs.[31]

In 1928 Dr. Abraham Myerson, a professor of neurology at Tufts College Medical School, published the first of a series of attacks on the scientific basis for diagnosing a genetic etiology in the feeble-minded.[32] This marked the start of a twenty-year crusade against eugenic sterilization programs. His attacks were always preceded by careful study. For example, in 1930 he published a study showing that the feeble-minded tended to come proportionately from all socio-economic classes rather than disproportionately from the poor, thus debunking another tenet of eugenics.[33]

In 1934, when the German sterilization program was initiated, the

American Neurological Association (ANA) appointed a committee chaired by Dr. Myerson to investigate commitment and sterilization patterns in institutions for the mentally ill. Supported by a grant from the Carnegie Institute (which, curiously, also funded Laughlin), the group worked full-time for a year; by June 1935, it had produced a 132-page report, which rejected virtually the entire eugenic thesis. Although the Myerson Report concluded that rates of institutionalization had risen steadily in America during the nineteenth century, the committee found no significant rise in the incidence of schizophrenia or manic-depressive illness during the first third of the century. Rather, the committee determined that the major reason for the vastly increased commitment rates was the availability of better medical care and improved hospital facilities. The major affliction suffered by most of the more recently admitted patients was "cerebral and arteriosclerotic psychoses" (senility), a consequence of the increasing life span. The committee noted that as hospitals improved, children "[did] not feel as if they [had] abandoned their parents to the lunatic asylum." It concluded that all the statistics "definitely indicate that there is no real increase in the commitment rate and that biologically, so far as mental disease is concerned, the race is not rapidly going to the dogs, as has been the favorite assertion for some time."[34]

The committee saw little benefit in sterilizing persons with mental impairment. It also advised against sterilizing normal persons known to be carriers of genes for severe genetic diseases (with the sole exception of Tay-Sachs disease). It found "no sound scientific basis for sterilization on account of immorality or character defect." It concluded that "environmental agencies of life" were often more influential than heredity. Rather than advocating that sterilization programs be ended, the Myerson Committee made three recommendations: programs must be wholly voluntary; enabling laws should apply to all persons, not just residents of state facilities; and sterilization recommendations should be made only by scientific experts.

The Myerson Report remains the definitive scientific critique of eugenic sterilization published in the United States. While the members clearly rejected compulsory sterilization, they did find it permissible if the patient or a guardian or family member consented to the surgery.

> Your Committee feels, in short, that it can only recommend sterilization in selected cases of certain diseases and with the consent of the patient or those responsible for him. We recommend that such selective sterilization be considered in cases of the following diseases (arranged roughly in the order in which sterilization would appear to be indicated):
>
> (1) Huntington's chorea, hereditary optic atrophy, familial cases of Fred-

rich's ataxia, and certain other disabling degenerative diseases thought
to be hereditary
(2) Feeble-mindedness of familial type
(3) Dementia praecox (schizophrenia)
(4) Manic depressive psychosis
(5) Epilepsy.[35]

The ANA report had an immediate political impact, and almost certainly torpedoed a sterilization bill in New York. On February 12, 1936, one eugenically minded New York legislator wrote to Dr. Clarence G. Campbell, president of the Eugenic Research Association, complaining, "All of a sudden, out of a clear sky comes the report of the American Neurological Society headed by Dr. Abraham Myerson of Boston and financed by the Carnegie Foundation, which says in substance that we do not know enough about heredity, environment and eugenics to decide whether compulsory sterilization is useful or not." The legislator warned that unless the report could be countered, "the sterilization bill will be dead in this state and probably all other movements to better the racial stock."[36] That same day, Judge Frank Cooper, a eugenicist who sat on the federal district court in Albany, sent a copy of the letter to Dr. Henry Perkins, president of the American Eugenics Society, asking that Perkins "kindly let me know what you think can be done to offset this Myerson report."[37] But the AES was unable to mount an effective counterattack.

In 1935 Myerson attacked Laughlin's model sterilization law in the pages of the *Archives of Neurology and Psychiatry*.[38] During the winter of 1936 he continued his campaign. On March 15, the *New York Times* published a long letter in which he dismissed pedigree studies like those of the Jukes and the Kallikaks as "mythical monstrosities," and urged that "the crying need of eugenics ... is not legislation, but real research."[39] When Macmillan published an enlarged version of the ANA report in 1936, Myerson included more data to refute the notion that the incidence of congenital mental retardation was rising. He also inserted a long review of twin studies that tended further to debunk a Mendelian etiology for most retardation.[40]

During 1934, the *Scientific American* devoted four articles to a debate over sterilization. Father J. H. Landman, a Jesuit lawyer-scientist, initiated the series with a powerful attack on the eugenicists. He characterized their theories as unproven and argued that behavioral conditioning and vocational training offered a better guarantee for a successful program of parole for the retarded than did sterilization.[41] In rebuttal a month later, Edwin Gosney summarized the studies in California, suggesting that sterilization benefited patient and society.[42] In September, the *Scientific American* published a second pro-sterilization article by a German physician named Thomalla that was an "officially sanctioned statement of Germany's aims in connection with racial and national eugenics." He argued that the German program was scientifically valid, economically sound, and ethically acceptable. Dr. Thomalla even asserted that compulsory sterilization was compatible with the tenets of Christianity.[43] The final article, by Ignatius Cox, professor of ethics at Fordham University and a leader of the Catholic critics, rejected sterilization on scientific, ethical, and political grounds.[44] The attention devoted by the *Scientific American* to this topic suggests that the new German program for a time made eugenics generally newsworthy to the American public.

The critique of eugenic sterilization produced by the American Neurological Association placed the Carnegie Institute in an unusual position. In 1935 it had funded both the Eugenics Record Office at Cold Spring Harbor and the ANA study that concluded that the pedigree studies carried on at the ERO were unscientific. In 1937 officials of the Carnegie Institute slashed funding for eugenic studies at Cold Spring Harbor, and in 1938 they informed Laughlin that "there are those who have not considered your work and your attitude, and perhaps your abilities, as representing the level of effectiveness which might be looked upon as the standard to be obtained in the Carnegie Institution."[45] Laughlin resigned the following year.

Despite the Myerson Report and other medical studies that debunked eugenic theories, the demise of the Eugenics Record Office, and vigorous Catholic opposition to new laws, sterilization programs remained active during the late 1930s. Each year hundreds of surgeons performed about two thousand vasectomies and salpingectomies on retarded persons in the name of social welfare. No laws were repealed and funding remained stable. It was one thing for a blue-ribbon group of neurologists to condemn eugenic sterilization in Boston and quite another to close the clinics at Lynchburg, Sonoma, and Faribault.

There is some evidence that the criticisms of Myerson and his contemporaries did little to reshape public attitudes. Consider a 1937 article in *Fortune*. Conducting its annual survey of reader opinions, the publisher asked: "Some people advocate compulsory sterilization of habitual criminals and mental defectives so that they will not have children to inherit their weaknesses. Would you approve of this?" Sixty-six percent of the respondents favored sterilizing mental defectives and 63 percent favored sterilizing criminals. Only 15 percent of the respondents were opposed. Given that by 1937 even most eugenicists acknowledged that a strictly hereditarian view of criminal behavior was untenable, the response is startling. Clearly, pro-sterilization views were widely held by the monied readers of *Fortune*.[46] Nor did the Myerson Report have much influence at the Girls' Industrial School, a correctional institute for teenagers in Beloit, Kansas. In 1937 the new superintendent was shocked to learn that 62 girls had recently been sterilized and that 22 operations were planned (which she promptly canceled). In its story about the exposé of the clandestine surgery, *Time* noted that Beloit was "front-page news throughout the U.S."[47]

Part of the explanation for the readers' responses to the *Fortune* question is that during the 1930s, pro-sterilization forces published a steady stream of propaganda. Perhaps the most radical propagandist of the era was Leon F. Whitney, whose book, *The Case for Sterilization*, argued that in order to protect the nation's biological future some ten million Americans should be sterilized as soon as possible. He conjectured that perhaps one-fourth of the entire population was unsuitable for parenthood. Whitney's zealous opinions were debunked even in the *Journal of Heredity*, but the book sold fairly well.[48]

The preeminent journalist of eugenics was unquestionably Albert Edward Wiggam. Starting around 1920, he produced scores of Sunday feature columns and several books that explained eugenics to millions of Americans. Careful about his facts, Wiggam frequently corresponded with (and soon befriended) Davenport, Laughlin, and other eugenicists. When his book *The New Decalogue of Science* appeared in 1922,[49] it won the praise of prominent eugenicists like G. Stanley Hall, president of Clark University.[50] Rarely making unreferenced statements, even in his popular books, Wiggam was an extremely effective propagandist. Thus, when he wrote that scientists had determined that "heredity is by all means" more important than environment in causing crime, his readers took heed.[51] Wiggam was adept at making sterilization sound like a blessing. He described the feeble-minded as "merely mental children," who should be "encouraged to set up homes and marry." They became a social danger only when they were "allowed to increase their numbers in a brood of children."[52]

It was during the 1940s that scientists opposed to involuntary sterilization really began to speak out. In 1946 two prominent geneticists, L. C. Dunn and Theodosius Dobzhansky, unequivocally rejected involuntary sterilization in their influential book, *Heredity, Race, and Society*.[53] But during the same period, Clarence Gamble, a Massachusetts physician, published at least twenty articles advocating sterilization. Writing in the *Journal of the American Medical Association* in 1949, Gamble described sterilization as "long range preventive medicine." He urged every physician to educate his patients so that "protection of the next generation from the inheritance of psychosis and mental deficiency will become more complete."[54]

The recent dramatic change in attitude toward the mentally retarded and the new emphasis placed on the possibility of helping many of them achieve a normal (noninstitutionalized, largely independent) life is beyond the scope of this book. The principle of "normalization" that emerged in the 1960s gave way to the more aggressive "rights" movement that exists today. Currently, some persons may wonder if the advocates of the mentally retarded have set unrealistic goals. But, when one understands that in the 1930s sterilization was sometimes the only "benefit" offered to a retarded person, it is clear that we have traveled a long way.

9 · The Quiet Years

The most significant development in eugenics after 1930 was its
rapid decline in popularity and prestige.
—Mark Haller, *Eugenics,* 1964

Do you favor forced sterilizations for mentally ill persons?
Yes—48%

—*Boston Globe,* reader survey, March 31, 1982

The 1930s saw the high water mark of eugenic sterilization in the
United States. During the 1940s and 1950s, a number of events forced the
movement into decline. The most important was the onset of World War
II. From 1942 through 1946, every available surgeon was in the armed
services. Those who stayed home had heavy practices, and eugenic sterilization programs were a low priority.

Opponents of involuntary sterilization spoke with a louder voice.
Geneticists, in particular, firmly rejected the eugenic thesis that feeble-
mindedness was a Mendelian disorder. The Catholic church, long opposed
to sterilization, remained a tireless critic. In 1942 the United States Supreme Court struck down an Oklahoma law that provided for the sterilization of thrice-convicted felons. Although the opinion in *Skinner v. Oklahoma* was decided on relatively narrow grounds and did not overrule *Buck
v. Bell,* it was a sign that the high court was breathing new life into the
Equal Protection Clause, and a warning that class legislation would be
carefully examined.[1] As the world grasped the full horror of Hitler, there
arose a new sensitivity to human rights issues. The 1940s engendered the
civil rights movement, with which involuntary sterilization programs were
incompatible.

Although these developments prevented the passage of sterilization
bills and slowed the rate at which surgery was performed, the programs
persisted. The decline that began with the onset of World War II was a
gradual one that lasted two decades and was by no means uniform. The

128

demise of the California program in 1952 was a major event, but sterilizations rose that year in a few states, notably North Carolina and Virginia.
As recently as the mid-1960s, long after most sterilization programs were
thought to have ended, a few states were still sterilizing several hundred
retarded persons each year.

The War Years

During the 1930s, about twenty-five hundred involuntary sterilizations were performed upon institutionalized persons each year. Some state
institutions and asylums had small operating suites, but many depended on
nearby hospitals to provide the facilities in which the surgery was performed. Although most state institutions had physicians, the rapid build-up
of the armed forces in early 1942 quickly thinned the staffs. The impact of
the war on eugenic sterilization programs was immediate, as replies to
surveys conducted during the war years indicate.

In 1941 Indiana officials arranged for the sterilization of 96 persons
in the state institutions, but at the close of 1942 the superintendent of
Central State Hospital in Indianapolis reported that the entire surgical staff
was in the service and no operations had been performed. Similarly, in
1944 the superintendent of Delaware State Hospital at Farnhurst reported,
"Because of the war situation and shortage of staff in our Mental Hygiene
Clinic, we have not been able to consider the problem of sterilization of
those who are at large."[2] In Kansas, where officials had been sterilizing
about 200 persons each year, the war caused a significant slump, which was
attributed to the reduced medical staff. The superintendent of Topeka State
Hospital reported that since losing his surgeon, there had been no sterilizations, but he hoped "to begin very shortly."[3] In Virginia, which from 1940
to 1942 led the nation in sterilizing institutionalized persons, there was a
precipitous drop from 332 in 1942 to 219 in 1943 and then to 131 in
1944, again owing to the shortage of surgeons. For the four-year period
from the start of 1941 through the end of 1944, 5,704 persons were
sterilized in the nation's institutions, an annual average of 1,426 which was
40 percent of the average number of operations performed annually during
the 1935-40 period. In 1945, only 1,336 sterilizations were performed.

The 1950s saw considerable public debate concerning whether it was
permissible to elect sterilization as a strategy to limit family size. Catholic
opposition to both eugenic and elective sterilization was sustained. In the
fall of 1953 Pope Pius XII, responding to a question put to him by representatives of an international conference on genetics, condemned eugenic sterilization and described the prohibition of marriage by persons

with hereditary taints as "morally contestable." The pope held that the morally irreproachable goal of preventing hereditary illness could not be achieved by forbidding the right to marry or by preventing procreation.[4]

In addition to the loss of surgeons to the armed services and the continued opposition of the Catholic church, the pace of sterilization programs may have been slowed by the United States Supreme Court decision in *Skinner v. Oklahoma*. At issue in *Skinner* was the constitutionality of Oklahoma's Habitual Criminal Sterilization Act, a law that had been enacted in 1935. Any person who was convicted of three felonies "involving moral turpitude" and who was thereafter confined to an Oklahoma penal institution was a potential subject for sterilization. The statute gave the state attorney general the power to institute proceedings to have the prisoner rendered sterile. The prisoner was afforded a jury trial, but the only question the jurors were to answer was whether he or she could be sterilized without detriment to his or her general health.

In 1926 a man named Skinner was convicted of stealing chickens; three years later he was convicted of armed robbery, and in 1935 he was confined on a third robbery conviction. In 1936 the attorney general filed a sterilization petition against him, and Skinner challenged its constitutionality. After the Supreme Court of Oklahoma upheld the law (5-4), he appealed.

The majority of the U.S. Supreme Court justices thought that a single glaring inequity made the statute unconstitutional. A special section of the law excluded persons convicted of several kinds of felonies (income tax evasion, embezzlement, and political offenses) from the reach of a sterilization petition. This meant, for example, that a person who was convicted on three occasions of stealing two hundred dollars by breaking and entering could be sterilized, but a bank clerk who was convicted of embezzling two hundred dollars by false bookkeeping practices on three occasions could not be sterilized. The majority opinion, written by William O. Douglas, held that the potential harm inherent in an involuntary sterilization law demanded "strict scrutiny" by the court of the reasoning by which a state chose to apply it to a selected class of persons. He recognized that "the power to sterilize, if exercised, may have subtle, far-reaching and devastating effects. In evil or reckless hands it can cause races or types which are inimical to the dominant group to wither and disappear." These words suggest that the German sterilization program had raised grave concern on the high court. Two justices wrote separate concurring opinions, but there was no dissenting vote in the decision to invalidate the Oklahoma statute.

Both Justice Douglas and Chief Justice Stone, who wrote one of the concurring opinions, cited the Myerson Report as a key source for their comments about the scientific validity of Oklahoma's statute. Although both expressed concern that the power to sterilize could be easily abused, Stone's words indicate that he believed some of the tenets of eugenics. For example, he wrote that "science has found and the law has recognized that there are certain types of mental deficiency associated with delinquency which are inheritable." He did, however, reject the possibility that "criminal tendencies of any class of habitual offenders are universally or even generally inheritable."

Skinner did not generate great public interest or commentary in academic circles. From 1943 through 1949, only one major law review article on involuntary sterilization was published. The Supreme Court ruling certainly precluded the enactment of other habitual criminal sterilization laws, but it did not alter existing policy in individual states regarding the sterilization of institutionalized noncriminal persons.

The Sterilization League of New Jersey

In the face of this rising tide of opposition, one reason why state programs favoring the eugenic sterilization of institutionalized persons did not decline even more quickly in the 1940s is that a few key advocates worked assiduously to sustain them. As had earlier been the case with the Eugenics Record Office and the Human Betterment Foundation, the New Jersey Sterilization League (NJSL) prospered thanks to the untiring efforts of a handful of people. The founder and key figure was Marion S. Norton, a social worker, a feminist, a virulent anti-Catholic, a woman of large vision and great tenacity, and a devoted advocate of the cause.[5]

Shortly after moving to New Jersey in the early 1930s, Mrs. Norton became active in the League of Women Voters, work that led to an invitation to start a "social hygiene department" for the local chapter. Mrs. Norton quickly developed a lecture series about public health problems. She drew on her experience with large, poverty-stricken families and her familiarity with the residents in the New Jersey state hospital to build pro-sterilization arguments. After a successful summer series, in the autumn she launched a more ambitious program that included field trips to most of the state institutions.

During 1935 Mrs. Norton led an effort by the League of Women Voters to draft a sterilization bill, collect signatures from physicians who favored it, and introduce it in the Senate. She also wrote a pamphlet advocating passage of the sterilization bill and organized exhibits at meetings like that of the New Jersey Conference on Social Work. Despite the league's work in favor of Senate Bill 50, the legislature did not give it serious consideration.[6]

In November 1936 Mrs. Norton, who had broken with the League of Women Voters when it rejected her more radical views, felt the time had come "to form a Sterilization League of New Jersey." The NJSL was born on March 20, 1937, with an initial membership of 23. The Honorable T. L. Zimmerman, a judge from Ridgewood, was named president. Despite a serious illness that summer, Mrs. Norton, who had been chosen as secretary, scored some remarkable successes. By the end of the first year she had enlisted 373 dues-paying members, raised thirteen hundred dollars, and developed an extensive slide show for her recruiting lectures.[7] By mid-1938 there were already signs that the Sterilization League was acquiring some political clout. In January Mrs. Norton gave a public lecture favoring sterilization of retarded persons before a large audience in Hackettstown. She so enraged the Catholic Knights of Columbus that it convened a special session to condemn the league and mailed a copy of the resolution to every lawmaker in the state. Mrs. Norton was undeterred. In December, for example, she spoke before the New Jersey Taxpayers Association on the budgetary savings that might be accomplished by a eugenic sterilization program.[8]

In 1939 Mrs. Norton persuaded her colleagues to draft another sterilization law. For two years the league and its lawyers repeatedly debated the issue, but by the end of 1941 the necessary compromises had been struck; in March 1942, a twenty-four-page bill to create a State Eugenic Commission was prepared. Since it was the pet project of twelve hundred influential citizens, the bill was rapidly put before the powerful Committee on Ways and Means. Entitled An Act to Aid the Afflicted by Providing for the Sexual Sterilization of Persons Unfit for Parenthood, the bill proposed hiring a "state eugenicist" to conduct a census of all persons in New Jersey to identify persons who were unfit for parenthood. It also recognized the right of noninstitutionalized persons likely to transmit a wide range of physical or mental defects to obtain elective sterilizations. Permission to be sterilized had first to be obtained from the state eugenicist.[9]

The bill immediately ran into serious political problems. Modeled partly after the German law, it empowered the state eugenicist to search all the state prisons, hospitals, homes, and asylums to find people "suffering from mental deficiency, familial mental disease, or family epilepsy and unable because of such affliction to discharge the responsibilities of parenthood." The eugenicist was to present sterilization petitions concerning such persons to a State Eugenic Council, which would hold hearings and decide each case. Patients were guaranteed a right of appeal, but if the courts ruled in favor of the finding, they could be sterilized despite their objections or the objections of their family.

The proposal to legalize eugenic sterilization angered New Jersey's Catholic leaders, and the bill's compulsory features provoked opposition from a broad group, including the League of Women Voters. One legislator warned Mrs. Norton that her proposal had become "a hot potato" about which, despite private feelings in its favor, most lawmakers "would not commit themselves." In due course the bill was referred to the Miscellaneous Business Committee, popularly known as "the morgue."[10]

This may have fostered the bitter struggle that soon swept the New Jersey Sterilization League. During late 1942 one faction sought to wrench control from Mrs. Norton, who ran it from her home in Princeton. Their plan was to move the headquarters to Newark, incorporate, and adopt a somewhat more moderate image. Mrs. Norton fought back. In January 1943 she prepared a press release castigating her opponents and threatened to quit.[11]

The threat worked; loyal co-workers came to her side, and a new plan of organization was developed that kept her in control. In April 1943, Marion S. Norton Olden (she had divorced and remarried) and a few colleagues founded Birthright, a nonprofit corporation with an avowed purpose to "devote itself primarily to a program of selective sterilization for those whose parenthood would violate *The Child's Bill of Rights* (which had been drafted by the White House Conference on Child Health and Protection in 1930). Birthright numbered several prominent leaders, including Robert Latou Dickinson, one of the nation's best-known obstetricians and a crusader for maternal health, and Professor E. A. Hooton, the Harvard anthropologist with strong ties to the eugenics movement.[12] Although Mrs. Olden was not elected to the original slate of officers, by 1945 she was the executive secretary and in control of daily operations.

In 1944 Birthright's power was significantly increased by the addition of a wealthy physician with staunchly eugenic views. Dr. Clarence Gamble, an heir to the Gamble soap fortune, wanted to expand vastly the use of eugenic sterilization programs. Dr. Dickinson persuaded Gamble that the most effective way for him to do so was to contribute to Birthright. But Gamble conditioned his financial aid on an agreement that Birthright create a research committee that he would control. Birthright agreed, and the Gamble Trust Fund in Cincinnati gave ten thousand dollars "for the educational work of the Field Committee." Dr. Gamble was even more zealous than Mrs. Olden. From the start she criticized his efforts to initiate sterilization programs at the grass-roots level, but he was undeterred. During the late 1940s Gamble traveled throughout the Midwest and South, starting more than twenty sterilization clinics in Michigan, Indiana, Iowa, Nebraska, Kansas, Missouri, and Florida.

His greatest success was in North Carolina, where in 1945 he paid for extensive intelligence testing of school-age children in Orange County. The results suggested that 3 percent of the population was mentally defective, a finding that Gamble used to press for the expansion of North Carolina's sterilization program. On June 16, 1945, the North Carolina Eugenics Board agreed to hire a sociologist (whose salary was paid by Gamble) to decide who in Orange County might benefit from sterilization. To counter the suspicions that some otherwise favorably disposed North Carolinians felt toward the northern-based Birthright, Gamble encouraged the founding of a local Human Betterment League of North Carolina, a strategy that had worked well in several other states.[13]

Despite his success, Mrs. Olden and her associates could not tolerate Gamble's independent style. On April 11, 1947, they resolved that his work "should no longer be carried out under the auspices of Birthright."[14] This led to a protracted struggle by Gamble to reclaim his ten thousand dollars, but it did not slow the pace of his North Carolina campaign. By helping to refocus eugenic sterilization from the state's institutions to the welfare rolls of each county, in three years Gamble more than doubled the number of eugenic sterilizations. During 1949 there were 249 sterilizations in North Carolina, second only to California.[15]

Despite his irritating ways, Gamble was a valuable asset and Birthright knew it. By 1949 he was back at work, although unrepentant and independently planning his local human betterment leagues. He also proved quite effective in publicizing the successes of the sterilization movement. His articles appeared in the *American Journal of Mental Deficiency* in 1947[16] and the *Journal of the American Medical Association* in 1949.[17] In both 1949 and 1950, *Newsweek* published favorable stories about Gamble's work.[18]

Birthright was repeatedly shaken by debate over whether it should adopt a more moderate course. Its long advocacy of involuntary sterilization had placed it in a position where Planned Parenthood and other organizations that were spearheading the larger birth control movement were leery of being identified with it. Mrs. Olden's strident attacks on the Catholic church also complicated potential alliances. During 1951 more moderate members of Birthright forced Olden and Gamble out of power and, under the leadership of Dr. H. Curtis Wood, formed the Human Betterment Association of America (HBBA). Although many of its members favored eugenic sterilization, the HBAA redirected its energies toward convincing the American public that elective sterilization should be used to limit family size, a goal it helped to accomplish in the 1960s and early 1970s.

Changing Patterns of Involuntary Sterilization (1945-1970)

With the demise of the Human Betterment Foundation after Gosney's death in 1942, the Sterilization League of New Jersey (and its successors) was the only organization conducting annual surveys of sterilization programs at the various state institutions. Despite frequent organizational changes and internal battles over policy, the league and its progeny continued these surveys until the mid-1960s. The responses of institutional officials to the survey questionnaires provide some insight into why eugenic sterilization gradually faded away.

During the postwar years, there was no immediate indication that the programs were going to decline. After hitting a low of 1,183 in 1944, the number of sterilizations climbed in 1945 and again in 1946, totaling 1,476 that year. A drop to 1,232 in 1947 was again followed by three consecutive increases. The 1,526 operations performed on institutionalized persons in 1950 fell far short of the nearly 2,500 a year that had occurred before the war, but were still substantial. Slight declines in most states and a sharp drop in a few (Minnesota, Michigan) were countered by rapid increases in North Carolina and Georgia.

There were, however, some signs that even in the most staunchly eugenic circles attitudes about sterilization were changing. During the late 1930s, many inmates (90 in 1938 and 145 in 1939) at California's San Quentin Prison agreed to be sterilized.[19] By 1947, however, the prison program had changed so significantly that prison officials would not even answer the survey questionnaire. Dr. Fred O. Butler, superintendent of the Sonoma State Home in Eldridge, California, managed to learn by telephoning a colleague at San Quentin in 1946 that only seven operations had been performed.[20] In April 1950 Dr. Stanley, the chief surgeon, informed Butler that only four vasectomies had been done in 1949, and observed that "the attitude of the present Department of Corrections is entirely adverse to sterilization," viewing it as a violation of prisoners' rights.[21]

In 1949 Birthright conducted a survey to determine how consent was obtained to sterilize institutionalized persons, virtually all of whom were not legally competent. The replies suggest that most programs made it a policy to obtain assent from a patient's relative. The view of what constituted assent varied widely. An Indiana official wrote that if a relative objected to the proposed sterilization, the institution did not press the matter in court. On the other hand, Georgia officials took a more aggressive approach. Parents of children for whom sterilization had been recommended were given just ten days to file a written protest, and failure to file an objection was considered an implied consent. Several years later, when Birthright repeated its survey of consent procedures, the replies suggested that because of growing doubts about eugenics, officials were adhering more closely to the procedural letter of the law. For example, an official at Eastern State Hospital in Williamsburg, Virginia, wrote that in addition to obtaining written approval from the designated state authorities, "the parents or legal guardian and patient are duly served with a notice of the proposed hearing and all provisions of the law are strictly observed."[22]

Concern for limiting the transmission of genetic disorders was fading in most states. In 1949 H. W. Hogan, a physician in charge of a sterilization program in South Dakota, commented, "We are further discovering that the so called heredity basis of feeblemindedness is becoming smaller, percentagewise, as the years go by." He thought that most cases were caused by encephalitis and birth injuries, and that sterilization was "by no means the answer to the problem." The medical superintendent of Missouri's Independence State Hospital reported that he only sterilized feeble-minded women whom he believed were sexually promiscuous, but that he did not sterilize persons to curb the flow of bad genes. Similarly, in 1956 J. M. Morris, the physician in charge of the Indiana Village of Epileptics, asserted that he did "not believe that epilepsy itself is sufficient reason for sterilizations."[23] This was in sharp contrast with the program in Lynchburg, Virginia, where many persons were then being sterilized because of epilepsy.

Survey responses in the late 1940s indicate that legislative interest in eugenic sterilization was much reduced. This may have been in part because several state attorneys general (Oklahoma, Mississippi) denounced their respective state laws as unconstitutional. Nevertheless, between 1945 and 1950 proponents of eugenic sterilization introduced bills in Alabama, New Jersey, Pennsylvania, and Idaho. While no new laws were enacted, neither were any repealed. Nor was there much judicial activity. Despite the suggestion in *Skinner v. Oklahoma* that courts might use the Equal Protection Clause to strike down some of the statutes, judicial struggles were waged and won by anti-sterilization forces only in two (Washington and Nebraska) of the thirty states with laws.

In 1949 Dr. Butler, who had presided over the sterilization of some five thousand mentally impaired patients in California over thirty years, became medical director of Birthright. As his first chore, he made an extensive national study of sterilization, traveling to thirty-four states and visiting nearly every institution that had an active program. His summary of that tour provides helpful evidence concerning public attitudes. He identified seven states where he thought that effective lobbying might still bring legislative victory: Arkansas, Alabama, Nevada, Kentucky, Washington, Tennessee, and New Jersey. Butler was aware that in Alabama and Arkansas there was "rising Catholic opposition," but he remained hopeful. In Kentucky, Nevada, and Tennessee he felt that pro-sterilization sentiment was strong and that a forceful leader could secure legislative victory. On the other hand, in Massachusetts, New York, Ohio, and Illinois he saw no hope for a law, largely owing to "strong religious opposition." Butler was also pessimistic about California, where Catholics had introduced a bill to restrict eugenic sterilization to cases in which the risk of transmitting a genetic disorder had been established in court. He concluded that of the twenty-one states with sterilization laws that he visited, thirteen were secure, but that in eight there was a need for Birthright to maintain a forceful propaganda effort.[24]

Butler focused Birthright's efforts on pointing out the potential savings that vigorous sterilization programs could mean for taxpayers. A press release issued by the Human Betterment League of Iowa in April 1949 is typical of material prepared by Butler. Its opening lines read: "Surgical sterilization has allowed feeble-minded patients in California 72,771 years of life outside of institutions since 1918 and saved the State $21,831,000, according to Dr. Fred O. Butler addressing the convention of the American Association of Mental Deficiency."[25]

Despite his medical training, there can be little doubt that Butler's strongly eugenic views blinded him to the difficulties inherent in deciding whether a patient would be helped by sterilization. A good example of his prejudice is found in his notes of a visit to an institution in South Carolina. He wrote that "when going through the buildings, it was obvious that many had both male and female patients who should be sterilized before leaving the institution."[26] Such clinical assessments can hardly be made with a glance.

The years 1949-51 saw two significant changes in eugenic sterilization programs. Most dramatic was the marked decline in California. In 1949 there had been 381 operations performed in California's institutions, but the number fell to 275 in 1950 and 150 in 1951; in 1952, only 39 operations were performed. As we have seen, these programs often depended on the attitudes of a few key people, and it is likely that the decline is most attributable to new officials at the California Department of Public Health who strongly opposed the practice. But events in California were countered by the expansion of sterilization programs in Georgia, North Carolina, and Virginia. In 1944 these states had been responsible for sterilizing 285 patients, or 24 percent of the nation's total. In 1952 they sterilized 673 patients, or 53 percent, and during 1958 they sterilized 574 patients, which constituted 76 percent of all reported operations.

The rise of sterilization programs in southern states does not appear to have been racially motivated. From its inception the Virginia sterilization program seems to have been applied about equally to both blacks and whites. In Petersburg State Colony, a black institution with 250 beds that opened in 1939, there were 137 sterilizations performed over the ensuing eight years. This number is similar to rates in comparable white institutions such as Lynchburg. Only in South Carolina, which operated a small sterilization program, is there strong evidence of racial discrimination. During 1954-55 South Carolina reported to Birthright that it sterilized 38 institutionalized persons. Of the 23 persons sterilized at the South Carolina State Hospital, an institution for the mentally ill of both races, all were Negro females.[27]

The rapid rise of state-supported sterilization in North Carolina is well documented. This program was unique in that it was not aimed solely at institutionalized persons. Although North Carolina had enacted sterilization laws in 1919 and 1929, the programs were small. In the years 1919-33, only 53 sterilizations were performed on institutionalized persons in North Carolina. After the enactment of a new law in 1933, a relatively large sterilization program was implemented. In 1934 there were 61 sterilizations, and in 1935 eugenic surgery was performed on 178 persons.[28]

The focus changed greatly in 1945, after state public health officials received the results of IQ tests conducted as part of a study of the rural poor that had been initiated by Clarence Gamble. They initiated a "voluntary" eugenic sterilization program in Orange County, hiring a professor of sociology from the University of North Carolina at Chapel Hill whose task was to identify persons who might benefit from sterilization and to educate them about its value. The Orange County program was quickly judged a success, and by 1948 welfare workers in many counties were searching for candidates for sterilization, a practice reminiscent of the tasks undertaken by ERO field workers before World War I. From 1948 through 1955 about 270 persons, half of whom were not residents of institutions, were sterilized annually. The majority (150) of the 186 patients operated upon in 1948 were poor women in rural counties.[29] As recently as 1963 the North Carolina Board of Eugenics paid the cost of sterilizing 193 persons, most of whom were poor young women living in the countryside.[30]

The success of the North Carolina program was partly due to lobbying by the Human Betterment League of North Carolina (an offshoot of Birthright), which frequently undertook mass mailing campaigns advocating sterilization. A typical letter read:

> Dear Friend:
>
> Last year in North Carolina more than 1200 children were born to feeble-minded parents. Others came into families of the insane. Many of these will inherit the mental handicap of their parents and all will be brought up in unsatisfactory surroundings.
>
> To prevent such tragedies in the future is one of the objectives of the Human Betterment League of North Carolina. When the average citizen knows that surgical sterilization
>
> (1) removes nothing from the body,
> (2) does not interfere with satisfactory married life,
> (3) makes no change in the patient except the desired one that children are not born, North Carolina's foresighted law for sterilization of the insane and the feeble-minded can be more adequately applied.
>
> Through widespread mailings of pamphlets, through lectures and meetings and through publicity in magazines and newspapers the League is informing North Carolina's public:
>
> (1) that the mental health of the next generation is of great importance,
> (2) that by sterilization the inheritance of mental handicap from the mentally diseased and defective can be prevented *without sacrifice,*
> (3) that by sterilization the future load on our State Hospitals and our Schools for the Feebleminded can be decreased as well as that of our Relief Funds and our *Taxpayers,*
> (4) that children can be spared the unhappiness of being reared by insane or feeble-minded parents. To expand this vital program for North Carolinians of this generation and the next we ask your contribution.[31]

A Human Betterment League also managed to increase eugenic sterilization in Iowa. From 1944 through 1947, there were about 50 sterilizations performed there each year. In 1947 the Iowa league, stimulated by events in North Carolina, began aggressively advocating eugenic sterilization of noninstitutionalized persons. In the next four years, despite "a higher proportion of Catholics and greater restriction of the discussion of things sexual," sterilizations tripled to an annual average of 145. With the demise of the league in Iowa in 1952, the annual number of operations dropped back to about 70.[32]

Faribault State Hospital

Little has been written about involuntary sterilization in the 1950s and 1960s. Knowledgeable persons, including physicians, geneticists, and mental health workers, have surmised incorrectly that by the late 1940s the practice of eugenic sterilization had virtually disappeared. To determine the extent to which sterilization was being quietly practiced, I explored the archives of several state institutions. In some states, such as Connecticut, I was unable to discover any evidence that eugenic sterilizations had ever been performed. However, at institutions in other states, such as the Faribault State Hospital in Minnesota, it was possible to trace sterilization policy from the 1930s to the present. Events there typified the period from 1945 to 1970.

Faribault State Hospital is a sprawling collection of institutional brick buildings that commands a lovely hillside fifty miles south of Minneapolis. In 1879 the legislature authorized the Board of Directors of the Minnesota Institute for the Deaf, Dumb and Blind to open a School for Feeble-Minded at Faribault. The progressive Minnesota citizens lured George H. Knight, whose father had founded just such an institution in Lakeville, Connecticut, thirty years earlier, to direct the new school.

The designation of the institution as a "school" reflects the optimism felt by the early students of mental retardation. By 1879, however, hope for educating the feeble-minded to become productive citizens in the world had given way to an emphasis on training them to function in a permanent custodial setting. At Faribault the notion that a school for the feeble-minded should be largely a self-sustaining asylum for lifelong residents flowered under the guidance of Dr. Arthur C. Rogers. From 1885 until his death in 1917, Rogers worked tirelessly to enrich the lives of his charges. He started a dairy farm, which they operated. There was a museum of natural history, a marching band that toured the state, annual outings by train to scenic spots, dances, burro rides, a factory for making brushes, and much vocational training. In 1906, when Dr. Walter Fernald, superintendent of a similar institution in Massachusetts, visited Faribault, he rated it among the best in the nation.[33] Today, one can still visit institutions such as the Templeton Colony in Massachusetts that were strongly influenced by Rogers's ideas.

Discussion of eugenic sterilization first rose at Faribault in 1897. In responding to a questionnaire concerning his views on surgical sterilization (in that era, castration), Rogers opposed parenthood for the feeble-minded but did not advocate preventive surgery. In 1899 he supported a bill prohibiting the marriage of feeble-minded persons, but in 1911 he opposed

Minnesota's first eugenic sterilization bill. This stance may have been more out of concern for adverse public reaction than opposition to the new, less mutilating vasectomy. After a bill authorizing the sterilization of "the feeble-minded, epileptics, rapists, certain criminal and other defectives" received some solid support in 1913, Rogers agreed to sit on a committee to prepare a model sterilization bill. Its recommendations were not implemented.[34]

During the 1920s, the Faribault staff strove to train some residents for community living. The Minnesota citizens who were then lobbying for a sterilization law argued that community placement enhanced the chances that retarded girls would become pregnant. A sterilization bill drafted by Dr. Charles Dight in 1924 failed, but in 1925 Dr. Frederick Kuhlman, director of the Division of Research of the Minnesota Board of Control, added his support, and a sterilization statute was adopted.[35]

The new law permitted the sterilization of feeble-minded and insane persons residing in state hospitals, but only after approval by a psychologist, a physician, the superintendent of the state school, and the State Board of Control. The statute also required consent by the patient or his or her legal representative. State officials promptly implemented a program, but given the procedural issues, it started slowly.[36] Only 21 persons were sterilized in the first half of 1926. After *Buck v. Bell* the pace quickened, and by the end of 1938, 1,280 persons had been sterilized at Faribault. Virtually all these operations were performed by Dr. George Eitel, a public-minded surgeon who worked there about two days a month.[37] A report written by E. J. Engberg, the superintendent during most of that era, confirms that Faribault was the only institution in the state at which the operation was performed, and that the policy was to sterilize only persons who were "considered suitable prospects for parole."[38] The sterilization program at Faribault was slowed, but not stopped, by World War II. Faribault's surgeons sterilized 273 persons between July 1, 1938, and June 30, 1940. By midsummer of 1942 there had been another 214 sterilizations, and by mid-1944 an additional 113 operations had been performed. However, in the next two years there were only 35 operations, and from 1946 through 1948 only 4 men were sterilized. According to the 1948 biennial report, a "shortage of nursing personnel prevented any more of the operations."[39]

In fact, something more than a nursing shortage caused the sharp decline. During a 1946 election campaign, some politicians charged that residents at Faribault were abused and subjected to wholesale sterilization. The newspapers made much of the charges, and not a few families of the residents expressed fear. A grand jury was convened, and it eventually concluded that the charges were unwarranted.[40] Nevertheless, the program became quiescent. During 1951 and 1952 there were only 17 sterilizations (15 women and 2 men). The 1954 biennial report acknowledges only 5 operations, and after that year no further sterilizations were reported. Mildred Thompson, a leading figure in the care of retarded persons in Minnesota, explained the change in this way:

> The success of wards in industry during the war had helped to bring about the change, perhaps somewhat unconsciously. If they were able to show greater ability and better judgment than we had expected, perhaps we need not be so concerned about the possibility of their having offspring. Moreover, some of the knowledge of human genetics gained during these later years had ended the idea that mental deficiency was inherited as an entity. Thus sterilization could be considered on a more selective basis.[41]

The fact that Faribault's biennial reports do not report sterilizations after 1954 does not mean that sterilizations ceased. Dr. Arthur Madow, a psychologist who began working there in the early 1950s and who in 1981 was program director at Faribault State Hospital, remembered that throughout the 1950s it was his job to conduct psychological testing of persons for whom sterilization was being considered, usually just prior to discharge. His records indicate that in the six years from 1955 through 1960 he examined 46 female and 8 male candidates for sterilization. Although he did not have records of the operations, he recalled that in most cases the candidates were sterilized.[42] According to Dr. Madow and to Dean Nelson, director of Social Services at Faribault, the sterilizations in the late 1950s were performed almost exclusively on mildly retarded young women who were leaving the institutions. A few were also performed upon noninstitutionalized retarded women who had given birth to illegitimate children. Mr. Nelson recalled that in that era, if a guardian refused to authorize sterilization, Faribault officials would not permit the woman to leave the institution.[43]

In 1961, eugenic sterilization at Faribault did stop. This change was coincident with the arrival of Dr. David Vail as director of the Medical Services Division of the Minnesota Department of Welfare. According to Dr. Madow, Dr. Vail was unequivocally opposed to eugenic sterilization, no matter how compelling the case.

By 1969, opposition was so strong that Faribault officials were unable to convince a judge of the wisdom of sterilizing a mildly retarded woman with five illegitimate children who had lost custody of them after repeated episodes of child abuse. Although he agreed with "the social desirability of the patient having no more children," the examining psychiatrist refused to recommend sterilization. He recommended that the woman be provided with birth control pills and that intensive therapy be directed at altering her behavior toward children. This, he asserted, was preferable to "infringing upon her civil rights through an intervening surgical procedure."[44]

In 1970, nine years after his arrival, Dr. Vail eased his policy against sterilization. His memorandum on the subject stated in part:

> In years gone by sterilizations were done rather often, especially on retarded persons, including males. In the past decade we have adopted a very conservative approach, and sterilizations are now quite infrequent. There are those who believe that the present policy is too strict, especially in the light of new knowledge about genetics and other recent developments.
>
> I think it is probably time to re-explore the question and examine the possibility of modifying the policy if a study indicates that this would be desirable.[45]

Between 1971 and 1975 Dr. Heinz Bruhl, medical director at Faribault, evaluated ten retarded women as candidates for sterilization. He approved nine of the applications and refused one on the grounds that the woman was probably already infertile.[46] But interest in sterilization continued to decline, and not more than one or two persons have been sterilized annually since then. Nevertheless, the evidence is clear that although very limited in scope, eugenic sterilization was quietly practiced at Faribault at least until 1975, nearly three decades after most people believe that such programs had ended.

Faribault is not an isolated case; a eugenic sterilization program was active in Iowa until as recently as 1976. That year the Jasper County Home in Iowa was closed by state officials after numerous allegations of violence toward patients. Among them was that officials had forced six young women to be sterilized as a condition of their discharge. Dr. Roy C. Sloan, the home's consulting psychiatrist, acknowledged that in the eight years he worked at Jasper sterilizations were routinely performed on young women, usually without any effort to obtain a legally valid consent. Since the State Board of Eugenics insisted that it approved sterilization *only* for the "severely mentally retarded" (179 operations between 1971 and 1976), the Jasper protocol clearly violated state policy. Less than a year after the scandal over Jasper County Home the legislature ended sterilizations at state institutions. The Jasper story demonstrates the persistence of sterilization programs despite the passing of the eugenic thesis.[47]

The Battle for Voluntary Sterilization

As eugenic sterilization programs were declining, the struggle to make elective sterilization an option for controlling family size was building. Of course, the birth control movement dates at least to the 1920s, when Margaret Sanger and her colleagues forced society to confront the fact that unwanted pregnancies constrained women's futures and endangered their lives. The debate has often divided along religious lines; Catholics and fundamentalists have opposed sterilization, while Protestants have supported an individual's right to choose. This was as true after World War II as it had been in 1930, when *Casti Cannubi* was published. For example, in 1947 the American Civil Liberties Union criticized the decision by officials in Catholic hospitals in Connecticut (a state where several crucial legal battles were fought) to expel non-Catholic physicians merely for supporting proposed legislation that would permit the use of birth control devices.[48]

On October 30, 1951, Pope Pius XII reaffirmed the Catholic doctrine prohibiting the use of contraception and added that the habitual use of the rhythm method was (except in special cases) a sin. His ringing reaffirmation of church doctrine elicited an upsurge in the political response of Catholic hospitals to the birth control movement. In January 1952, officials at St. Francis Hospital in Poughkeepsie, New York, ordered non-Catholic physicians to sever their ties with the local chapter of Planned Parenthood or lose their staff privileges.[49]

As patients and physicians became less secretive about their use of elective sterilization, the issue was more regularly litigated. One early legal victory for birth control advocates occurred in Richmond, Virginia, in 1952 when a jury found in favor of a physician who had sterilized a woman with four children without first obtaining the written consent of her husband.[50] The case received significant attention in medical journals, and it generated many questions among physicians. At that time there were no statutes clarifying an individual's right to be sterilized. Legal scholars usually advised that because sterilization had not been expressly prohibited, it could (assuming the patient had consented) be performed. Even so, lawyers took a most cautious approach. For example, as recently as 1959, Greenbaum, Wolff and Ernst, a New York law firm that represented birth control advocates, advised, "There is little doubt that were a case to come to court, the Judge would view the surgeon's case more favorably if the operation appeared as a therapeutic rather than a purely contraceptive operation."[51]

By 1960 the number of surgeons willing to perform elective sterilizations had grown significantly. The cause received an important boost in

April of that year when an article in the *Bulletin* of the American College of Surgeons reported that the thirty-five insurance companies writing malpractice policies would defend lawsuits growing out of the disputes over sterilization.[52] Nevertheless, hospital authorities remained cautious. In December 1961 the Joint Commission on Accreditation of Hospitals noted that most of their members permitted sterilizations "for pathological reasons only," and advised that written consent of the patient and his or her spouse should be obtained.[53]

Pressure for access to elective sterilization grew steadily. During 1960, the Human Betterment Association of America (HBAA) received 2,567 requests for advice on where to obtain surgery. In 1961, the Virginia State Medical Society lobbied successfully for a law protecting physicians from any liability in connection with a properly performed elective sterilization. In May 1962, Ruth Proskauer Smith, the daughter of a prominent New York Judge and the director of the HBAA, offered to pay for a sterilization clinic in Fayette County, Kentucky, an area with much poverty. County officials rejected her proposal.[54]

In 1962 the nation's attention was suddenly riveted on the issue. On September 3, the HBAA invited twenty sociologists attending a convention in Washington, D.C., to visit a family planning clinic at the Fauquier (Virginia) County Hospital, where fifty indigent women had been sterilized over the last two years. Sterilization was offered only to women who had had three children, was performed only after obtaining the consent of the patient and her husband, and was preceded by a thirty-day waiting period. A follow-up survey of the patients reported that only one regretted her choice. The *Washington Post* carried a story on the Fauquier program, and within days there was a national debate.[55]

Patrick O'Boyle, archbishop of Washington, preached a sermon denouncing the program as immoral. He accused the hospital of the "crudely selfish and materialistic" goal of reducing the tax rate. Noting the high proportion of Negro patients (two-thirds), he charged the clinic with racism.[56] A day later, evangelist Billy Graham joined the archbishop in condemning the elective sterilization of indigent women. In response, the HBAA pointed out that the National Council of Churches had approved sterilization as a means of limiting family size.

On September 12, the *New York Times* ran a story on the Fauquier debate that was generally supportive.[57] By September 24, when *U.S. News and World Report* carried a long article, the tide seemed to be favoring proponents of elective sterilization. The article quoted the Reverend William Genne, director of the Department of Family Life of the National Council of Churches, as saying that the Protestant faith recognized the freedom of an individual to choose sterilization. It also reported that Fauquier Hospital had been inundated by calls from many other hospitals that were seeking to start similar programs.[58]

During 1963 and 1964 the activities of the HBAA, Planned Parenthood, and other groups accelerated. Heady with the success in Fauquier County, the Human Betterment Association for Voluntary Sterilization (as the HBAA was renamed) opened new programs in Appalachia. In July 1964, it won a major victory when Jesse Hartman, a wealthy New York businessman, contributed twenty-five thousand dollars to help indigent patients obtain elective sterilizations in Kentucky.[59] A few months later he gave another twenty-five thousand to launch sterilization programs in several poor Florida counties. The widespread publicity attending these developments may have stimulated interest among state legislators in passing laws to legalize the right of a person to be sterilized.

There were the inevitable anecdotes about abuse. For example, in April 1963, a North Carolina judge who had found a mother of three illegitimate children guilty of neglect allegedly told her that she could avoid prison by submitting to sterilization.[60] Not infrequently, legislators muddied the debate by proposing to condition grants of state aid to welfare mothers upon proof of sterility. A few legislators even suggested punishing prostitutes by sterilizing them, suggestions that recalled the eugenic themes of earlier decades.[61] Part of the hesitation with which citizens greeted elective sterilization was probably due to its historic association with programs to curb reproduction by the feeble-minded.

As the 1960s progressed and the United States Supreme Court issued a series of rulings that upheld the individual's right to use birth control, the number of sterilizations mushroomed. Yet, as recently as 1970, in many states it was relatively difficult for a person to obtain an elective sterilization. This stimulated the Association for Voluntary Sterilization (the HBAA again renamed) to join with Zero Population Growth (ZPG) and the American Civil Liberties Union to launch Operation Lawsuit.[62]

Beginning in 1970, when Janet Stein, a twenty-seven-year-old mother of three, sued a hospital in Mr. Kisco, New York, claiming $250,000 in damages owing to its refusal to allow their facilities to be used for her elective sterilization, suits sprouted up quickly. Irate women sued hospitals in New York City; Salt Lake City; Eugene, Oregon; Tucson; and Highland Park, Michigan. The Michigan case was of special importance because the plaintiff attacked the spousal consent requirement. By mid-1971, ZPG chapters throughout America were recruiting plaintiffs for sterilization litigation. They had acquired such power that Catholic hospital officials often chose to negotiate a compromise with them rather than risk losing a lawsuit. At the end of 1971, the pro-sterilization coalition was involved in twelve lawsuits against hospitals.[63]

Throughout the early 1970s, in part due to the work of Jeremiah S. Gutman, a member of the New York Civil Liberties Union, many of these cases were aggressively litigated. So successful were they that the ACLU frequently was able to get hospitals to liberalize their rules merely by suggesting the possibility of a lawsuit. The victory was sealed in January 1973, when the United States Supreme Court decided *Roe v. Wade*.[64] This historic opinion, which held that a woman's constitutionally protected right to privacy included the right to obtain an abortion, ended the legal struggle over sterilization. A concept of privacy broad enough to encompass the termination of a pregnancy was surely broad enough to encompass less dramatic interventions.

10 · Involuntary Sterilization Today

"Court Refuses to Order Hearing on Sterilization."
—*Houston Post*, March 12, 1981

"Proposal for Woman's Sterilization Draws Protest."
—*New York Times*, September 25, 1988

During the 1950s and 1960s, institutionally based sterilization programs ended in many states and diminished in the rest. But the laws that
created them remained. After a thorough review in 1961, the American Bar
Foundation concluded that it was still legally possible to perform involuntary eugenic sterilizations in twenty-six states and that in six the law's
reach theoretically extended to all citizens.[1]

At least five states (Kansas, Indiana, Nebraska, North Dakota, and
South Dakota) have since repealed their sterilization laws. But even at the
height of the civil rights era, six states (Connecticut, Maine, Minnesota,
Montana, North Carolina, and West Virginia) chose to amend rather than
to abolish their laws. As recently as 1975, West Virginia enacted a sterilization law. Writing favorably about it, one West Virginia lawyer noted that
3,475 persons resided in the state's institutions for the mentally retarded
and, echoing Laughlin and Butler, asserted that eugenic sterilization was a
tax-saving measure.[2]

During the 1970s, a few states forbade involuntary sterilization of the
mentally retarded. In 1977, New Jersey outlawed the sterilization of the
"developmentally disabled at any facility" without the express and informed consent of the individual or his or her guardian. In 1979 California
and the District of Columbia banned the sterilization of any person under
the government's care. But as recently as 1985, at least nineteen states had
laws that permitted the sterilization of mentally retarded persons (Arkansas, Colorado, Connecticut, Delaware, Georgia, Idaho, Kentucky, Maine,
Minnesota, Mississippi, Montana, North Carolina, Oklahoma, Oregon,
South Carolina, Utah, Vermont, Virginia, and West Virginia).

During the 1960s, a new kind of sterilization lawsuit emerged: courts were petitioned to approve the sterilization of noninstitutionalized retarded women. In 1968, a Kentucky court refused to grant a declaratory judgment to permit a county health official to sterilize a thirty-five-year-old retarded woman with two children.[3] Similarly, in 1969 a Texas court refused to permit the mother of a thirty-four-year-old noninstitutionalized, retarded woman who had given birth to two retarded children to have her daughter sterilized. The Texas decision, *Frazier v. Levi,* was the first of a series of cases in which judges refused to grant sterilization petitions pertaining to noninstitutionalized persons without specific enabling legislation.[4]

During the late 1960s and the 1970s, the consensus among interested legal scholars was that the eugenic sterilization laws were no longer constitutionally valid, but the outcome of the few legal assaults on these statutes does not support this. Consider a 1968 challenge to the Nebraska statute. Gloria Cavitt, a mother of eight illegitimate children, had been committed to the Beatrice State Home for the retarded. On IQ testing she scored 71 and was labeled as mildly retarded. The Nebraska statute required that retarded persons be sterilized before being discharged, and in accordance with that rule the superintendent filed a sterilization petition. The patient promptly challenged the law.

By a vote of 3-4 (in Nebraska no statute could be declared unconstitutional without 5 concurring votes, so a minority of 3 could control the outcome) the law was upheld. Three months later, in an identical vote, the court denied a motion to reconsider the case. Of particular interest is the reasoning of the three justices who considered the statute constitutionally valid. They wrote: "The order does not require her sterilization. It does provide, in accordance with the statute, that she shall not be released unless she is sterilized. *The choice is hers*" (emphasis by the court).[5] To assert that a patient whose release from a state institution is contingent upon submitting to surgery nevertheless has freedom of choice mocks the principle. Not surprisingly, *In re Cavitt* was greeted with a storm of criticism, and the Nebraska legislature repealed the sterilization law at its next session. Still, it had survived constitutional challenge.

Eight years later (1976), a United States District Court in Raleigh, North Carolina, upheld the constitutionality of that state's law, one that permitted the county directors of social services to institute sterilization proceedings against noninstitutionalized persons under certain circumstances. In reaching its decision, the court noted that between June 1970 and April 1974, twenty-three persons had been sterilized—further evidence of the dogged persistence of these programs.[6]

In December 1973, the United States District Court in Alabama reached a decision that contrasted markedly with the North Carolina case and that heralded a new level of scrutiny of proposals to sterilize institutionalized persons. Earlier that year, a woman in Tuscaloosa who was the aunt and legal guardian of Ricky Wyatt, a resident of the Partlow State School, filed a lawsuit attacking the constitutionality of the Alabama eugenic sterilization law, which permitted officials at Partlow to decide whether to "sterilize any inmate." The three sitting federal judges held that by giving the power to sterilize to the "unfettered discretion" of two officials, the law violated the most basic requirement of due process, and was thus unconstitutional.

In defending their sterilization program, Partlow officials cleverly argued that they "never relied" on the statute as authority for performing the operations, depending instead on the consent of the individual's family. This meant that striking down the statute did not automatically protect the residents. Chief Judge John Johnson decided that this could only be accomplished by issuing an order that precisely defined the procedures that Partlow officials had to meet before they could contemplate eugenic sterilization. He prohibited the sterilization of any inmate unless there had been a prior determination "that no temporary measure for birth control" would meet the needs of that inmate. He also forbade predicating the decision to sterilize on "institutional conveniences." Further, no person under the age of twenty-one was to be sterilized except for "medical necessity." Johnson also required that, where possible, the resident be asked to execute a written informed consent. The consent would be considered "informed" only when it was secured after thorough efforts to explain the procedure in a climate unclouded by coercion. If the inmate was adjudged "legally incompetent" or if the superintendent was unwilling to state that the individual understood the nature of the proposed sterilization, the operation could be performed only if a special review committee approved it *and* a court subsequently agreed that it was in the best interest of the resident. The review committee (which had to include a physician, an attorney, two women, two minority group members, and at least one other resident of Partlow) was to follow strict procedural guidelines. This included review of appropriate "medical, social and psychological" information and interviews with the resident. Further, the individual had to be represented by an attorney. Finally, the judge required that written records be kept of all deliberations.[7]

In 1973 a widely publicized scandal concerning an Alabama physician who was accused of sterilizing black teenage girls without their consent resulted in an unprecedented level of judicial review of federally supported family planning clinics. Although this case did not involve institutionalized persons, the victims seemed nearly as powerless. The wire services reported that a surgeon at an HEW-funded clinic had sterilized four young sisters without their consent. Joseph Levin, the attorney for the young women, later acknowledged that there were only two sisters and that only one (a twelve-year-old mildly retarded girl named Minnie Relf) was sterilized.[8] On July 31, 1973, she and the National Welfare Rights Organization (NWRO) filed a class action lawsuit to ban the use of federal funds for any sterilization.

Within weeks the Department of Health, Education and Welfare announced its first "Notice of Guidelines for Sterilization under HEW Supported Programs," guidelines intended to protect "minors and other legally incompetent individuals" receiving services in federally funded clinics. Although the Family Planning Services and Population Research Act of 1970 (which supported such clinics) had not addressed sterilization, the secretary of HEW had defined sterilization as a contraceptive option that should be made available through the programs operated under this law.

As the *Relf* case was being litigated, HEW continued to develop its sterilization guidelines. On February 6, 1974, HEW issued final regulations, which the NWRO promptly attacked. The disputed regulations covered four classes of persons. They required that legally competent adults could be sterilized only after signing a written informed consent that acknowledged that the decision not to be sterilized would incur no loss of federal benefits. For legally competent persons under the age of eighteen (such as young married women or men), the regulations required that a review committee determine if the proposed sterilization would be in the patient's best interests. For legally incompetent minors, the regulations conditioned sterilization upon prior judicial review. Finally, concerning the sterilization of mental incompetents of any age, sterilization would be permitted only after the approval of the individual's representative and the review committee.

On March 15, 1974, the United States District Court for the District of Columbia struck down the HEW regulations. Judge Gerhart Gesell ruled that HEW had no authority to provide sterilization services to "any person incompetent under state law to consent to such an operation, whether because of minority or mental deficiency." Further, he ruled that sterilizations could only be paid for with federal funds in circumstances in which competent persons gave a "voluntary, knowing and uncoerced consent."[9] HEW appealed and the Court of Appeals returned the case to Judge Gesell, directing him to review new regulations that the government had quickly proposed. Gesell again rejected them. He did not think that HEW was "sufficiently funded to enable it systematically to monitor individual decisions to sterilize."[10] In April of 1974 HEW published "interim regulations" that placed even more restrictions on the use of federal funds for sterilization than Gesell had required. These interim regulations remained in effect throughout the judicial proceedings. The matter was finally resolved when the Court of Appeals, learning that no plaintiff had objections to the interim regulations and that they would remain in effect until HEW completed a new rule-making plan, declared the matter closed.[11]

On November 8, 1978, HEW published "final rules" on sterilizations performed under programs receiving financial assistance from the federal government (Medicaid, Title XX Social Services Programs, AFDC, and programs administered by the Public Health Service). The rules prohibited the use of federal funds to sterilize persons under age twenty-one, mentally incompetent persons of any age, and institutionalized persons of any age. In addition, the regulations required that any individual who wished to be sterilized must sign a special consent form and wait thirty days before undergoing the operation. To obtain a valid consent, the person educating the patient was required to offer to answer any questions, advise the person that he or she was free to withdraw consent any time before the sterilization without affecting his or her access to benefits, describe alternate methods of family planning, advise that sterilization was irreversible, give a thorough explanation of the procedure, including its discomforts and risks, explain the benefits of the procedure, and discuss the waiting period. If the potential patient did not understand English, an interpreter was required. If the individual was blind, deaf, or otherwise handicapped, other suitable arrangements to ensure adequate communication were mandatory. The individual also was given the right to have a witness present. Further, the rules prohibited efforts to obtain consent when the individual was in labor, seeking an abortion, or under the influence of alcohol or drugs. The federal guidelines introduced a new standard for reviewing the sterilization of the mildly retarded, the mentally ill, the uneducated, and the poor.[12]

The Retarded and the Right to Be Sterilized

Although legal scholars assert that *Buck v. Bell* is no longer "good" law, it has never been overturned, and the few courts that have considered the constitutionality of involuntary sterilization statutes have upheld them. In 1972 an Oregon court heard an appeal by a seventeen-year-old girl with a history of severe emotional disturbances and "indiscriminate and impulsive sexual involvements" from a sterilization order issued by the State Board of Social Protection. In upholding the order, the court explicitly relied on *Buck v. Bell,* concluding that "the state's concern for the welfare of its citizenry extends to further generations and where there is overwhelming evidence, as there is here, that a potential parent will be unable to provide a proper environment for a child because of his own mental illness or mental retardation, the state has sufficient interest to order sterilization."[13] Four years later, the Supreme Court of North Carolina also relied on *Buck v. Bell* in rejecting a similar attack on its sterilization statute. It disagreed with the plaintiffs' argument that to approve a sterilization there must be clear and convincing evidence (a higher than usual standard) that the operation would benefit the patient.[14]

Recent litigation has focused on articulating the right of retarded persons to be sterilized. Most of the suits have sought to determine whether judges have the power, lacking specific statutory authority, to order sterilization and/or to articulate the criteria by which such decisions should be made. Also, as federal guidelines have become more restrictive, some persons have criticized them as overly protective. They have argued that there is a right to be sterilized, that it can be asserted on behalf of another, and that it is wrong to limit severely the exercise of that right just because a person is a member of an "at-risk" group. In 1976 several New York surgeons joined with their poor patients to attack the regulations that refused under any circumstances to pay for the sterilization of a legally incompetent person. Their opponents countered that it was impossible for welfare recipients to exercise a truly voluntary choice in matters having to do with reproduction; therefore, it was better to shield them from coercion.

By 1979 there was apparent concern that the law deprived retarded persons of a significant therapeutic choice. As two physicians wrote: "Current law and rulings in seeking to protect the retarded as a group do major disservice to the severely handicapped. Cumbersome legal procedures, while avoiding the rare abuse, place sterilization beyond their reach. There is clear need to recognize that the retarded are not homogeneous and that decisions regarding sterilization and hysterectomy must be individualized."[15]

Many courts have since been asked to approve sterilizations for young, noninstitutionalized retarded (usually female) persons. This has largely been because of the surgeons' understandable reluctance to sterilize retarded persons without an explicit guarantee that they would not be violating the law. The cases, which are typically filed by parents who are caring for their retarded children at home, have provoked considerable debate over whether to permit such sterilizations.

In at least six states (Missouri, Indiana, California, Delaware, Alabama, and Maryland), courts have ruled that, without express statutory direction to do so, they could not order the sterilization of a retarded person.[16] An unusual 1977 decision by a federal appellate court holding that a judge who had approved the sterilization of a fifteen-year-old "somewhat retarded" female could be sued for acting in excess of his jurisdiction undoubtedly influenced judges who heard petitions after that. The case, *Sparkman v. McFarlin,* arose when a young woman who had been sterilized without her consent (she was told that she needed an appendectomy) learned of her infertility. She successfully sued her mother, who had requested the operation; the physicians who performed it; and the judge who had approved it.[17] While *Sparkman* was under appeal, state courts were reluctant to approve similar sterilization petitions.[18] In 1978 the United States Supreme Court reversed the appellate court, reasserting the important principle of judicial immunity. The high court did not comment on the judge's questionable behavior (he had ordered sterilization without even holding an evidentiary hearing), nor did it seize the opportunity to overturn *Buck v. Bell,* instead limiting its opinion to protecting the doctrine of judicial immunity.[19]

Since the early 1970s, the highest courts in at least nine states (Alabama, Alaska, Colorado, Massachusetts, New Hampshire, New Jersey, Vermont, Washington, and Wisconsin) have heard cases that have forced them to decide whether they have the power to approve petitions to sterilize retarded persons and, if so, to determine the criteria by which such petitions will be judged. The cases have often involved struggles between parents of a young retarded woman who resolutely believe that their daughter would be harmed by pregnancy and hospitals fearful that in providing the sought-for service they will be violating the retarded person's rights. Advocacy groups have occasionally played a key role. In Vermont the American Civil Liberties Union convinced a court that in seeking sterilization, parents of retarded children living at home must adhere to the same procedural guidelines as those created to protect institutionalized persons.[20] Parents of three profoundly retarded girls in Connecticut succeeded in obtaining an order to the University of Connecticut Health Center to perform hysterectomies.[21] In issuing the order, the federal district court opined that to provide institutionalized persons with access to sterilization without providing the same service to noninstitutionalized persons was a violation of the Equal Protection Clause.

During the 1980s the supreme courts in Alaska, Colorado, Massachusetts, New Hampshire, New Jersey, Washington, and Wisconsin ruled that lower courts of general jurisdiction have the power to decide sterilization petitions. The high courts have also usually articulated standards to guide the lower courts in passing upon such petitions. The New Jersey Supreme Court issued the leading opinion in this area. Lee Ann Grady, a young woman with Down syndrome, had always lived at home with her parents. When she reached adolescence and became interested in boys, her parents, fearful that she would be raped or seduced, started her on birth control pills. As she approached the age when she would leave school and enter a sheltered workshop, her parents, concerned about her safety, asked their physician to sterilize her. The local hospital refused to permit the operation, and the Gradys asked the court to authorize sterilization. After the judge ruled in favor of the operation, the attorney general appealed to the New Jersey Supreme Court.

There was little doubt that the Supreme Court, the court that had authorized the father of Karen Ann Quinlan to exercise by proxy her right to refuse extraordinary medical care, would recognize that the judiciary had the power to order sterilizations. Yet the *Grady* court did depart substantially from the *Quinlan* decision. In *Quinlan* the awesome choice of terminating extraordinary life support measures for incompetent (comatose) persons had been left to the family and physicians. But in *Grady* the court held that the sterilization of a retarded person would always require judicial approval. In commenting upon its departure from *Quinlan,* the court noted that sterilization of the mentally impaired had a "sordid history" of abuse.

The New Jersey attorney general had argued that sterilization should be limited to those cases where it could be shown that the person was likely to be sexually active and that other means of contraception would not work. The court refused to apply such a standard, understandably fearing that it might create a situation where a pregnancy must precede sterilization. It did, however, establish strict guidelines to protect the party on whose behalf sterilization was sought. It required the appointment of a guardian to represent the retarded person, evaluation by independent medical experts, and a personal meeting between the judge and the individual to discuss sterilization. The high court made clear that a judge should not approve a sterilization unless he or she decided that the individual herself (I know of no cases involving men) permanently lacked the capacity to exercise such a choice. It also ruled that the judge must be persuaded by clear and convincing evidence that sterilization would be in the person's best interest. Nine factors had to be considered in determining this issue: the possibility of becoming pregnant, the possibility that pregnancy would cause psychological damage, the likelihood that the individual would voluntarily engage in sexual activity, the inability to understand reproduction or contraception, the feasibility of other means of contraception, the advisability of sterilization now rather than later, the ability to care for a child, the likelihood of therapeutic advances that would improve the underlying condition or alter the need for sterilization, and a demonstration of good faith on the part of the proponents of the sterilization. *Grady* has guided the reasoning of a number of courts faced with similar questions.[22]

Poe v. Lynchburg

On December 29, 1980, the American Civil Liberties Union, acting on behalf of five plaintiffs and all living persons who had been operated upon under Virginia's eugenic sterilization statute between 1924 and 1974 (when it was repealed), filed a suit, *Poe v. Lynchburg,* against the various institutions where those operations had been performed.[23] The story of Judith Doe, the pseudonym of one plaintiff, a middle-aged woman who was sterilized at the Lynchburg Training School in 1949 (when she was fourteen) is typical. She alleged that she was admitted to Lynchburg shortly after she gave birth to a son who was conceived when she was raped by her stepfather. At Lynchburg she was told that she needed to have her appendix removed and that she could not leave the hospital unless she submitted to surgery. Judith was not given psychological or intelligence tests prior to the operation, and the Lynchburg records merely indicate that she was not thought to be "defective." She was discharged shortly after recovering from her "appendectomy." A few years later Judith married; her subsequent divorce, she alleged, was due to the inability to have children.

According to an attorney for the plaintiffs, the results of pretrial investigations indicated "that many individuals were not told that the operation would result in depriving them of the ability to have children, that the guardians appointed for the individual patients did not participate actively in the hearings to protect their clients, and that other procedural and substantive safeguards were not afforded to the sterilized individuals."[24]

In *Poe* the plaintiffs sought four things: a declaration that the involuntary surgical sterilization of institutionalized persons had violated the Due Process Clause of the Fourteenth Amendment, a declaration that the continuing failure to notify persons who were sterilized of that fact and of the possibility of surgically reestablishing their fertility also violated the right to due process, an order enjoining the defendants from conducting any further sterilization without obtaining informed consent, and an order requiring that all persons sterilized under the law be notified of their status and offered "medical, surgical and psychological assistance." Because the lawsuit attacked actions taken under a state law that had been upheld by the United States Supreme Court in *Buck v. Bell,* the defendants brought a motion to dismiss. In April 1981, Chief Judge Turk of the United States District Court for Western Virginia threw out the portions of the complaint that attacked the constitutionality of the original sterilization law, but decided to hear arguments as to whether a continuing failure to notify persons who had been unknowingly sterilized of that fact constituted a violation of their civil rights.

Poe v. Lynchburg stimulated the most in-depth study of sterilization in a single state since Gosney and Popenoe studied California's program in the late 1920s. The governor himself issued the order to the Department of Mental Health and Mental Retardation to compile and publish data on the number of persons who had been sterilized.[25] The data shown in table 8 cover the period from 1924 through 1979 (since 1973, sterilizations of persons in Virginia institutions have been permitted only for reasons of medical necessity). Remarkably, the survey revealed that the number of operations did not appreciably diminish until 1961, and that the program was reasonably active in the mid-1960s.

A settlement agreement between the class action plaintiffs and the state of Virginia was reached in 1983. Under its terms the state agreed to attempt to identify and inform all persons who were sterilized while under institutional care of that fact and to provide them with modest compensation.

The Etiology of Mental Retardation

Eugenic sterilization programs were implemented upon the premise that most mental retardation is inherited. In the early part of this century, thanks largely to the influence of Charles Davenport, mental retardation was thought to be the result of Mendelian disorders, the product of a defect in a single gene or pair of genes. By the 1930s, as it became clear that in many affected families the history of a disorder did not obey Mendel's laws, hereditarians began to postulate that the interaction of several genes was responsible. We still have much to learn about the causes of the hundreds of disorders that are collectively termed mental illness and mental retardation. But today our understanding has advanced sufficiently that we can address the concerns of Davenport and the eugenicists.

Mental retardation is generally classified as mild, moderate, severe, or profound. Each of these categories may be roughly described as comprising individuals whose intelligence testing falls in a specific region of the testing scale: mild, 55-69; moderate, 45-54; severe, 30-44; profound, 0-29. About 90 percent of all retarded persons are mildly retarded, and it is virtually certain that the vast majority of persons who were sterilized were either

Table 8 Involuntary Sterilizations in Virginia Institutions, 1924-1979

Year	All Hospitals	Central	Eastern	Southwestern	Western	Lynchburg	Petersburg
1979	2	0	0	0	0	2	0
1978	2	0	0	0	0	2	0
1977	3	0	0	0	0	3	0
1976	1	0	0	0	0	1	0
1975	4	0	0	0	0	4	0
1974	3	0	0	0	0	3	0
1973	8	0	4	0	0	4	0
1972	2	0	0	0	0	2	0
1971	6	0	6	0	0	0	0
1970	11	3	4	0	0	6	0
1969	22	7	7	0	2	6	0
1968	9	4	3	0	0	2	0
1967	16	9	2	0	1	4	0
1966	23	6	1	0	2	14	0
1965	28	2	2	2	2	21	0
1964	23	15	0	2	3	3	0
1963	38	10	0	9	5	14	0
1962	28	9	2	6	6	5	0
1961	17	12	1	10	6	2	0
1960	97	7	2	17	30	27	0
1959	76	19	9	· 2	16	11	19
1958	110	23	2	12	42	17	14
1957	113	59	4	0	26	24	0
1956	87	16	4	10	37	20	0
1955	80	23	4	0	39	44	0
1954	195	43	19	0	35	55	13
1953	176	55	6	12	23	82	0
1952	152	40	5	0	34	65	6
1951	201	44	18	1	58	78	2
1950	228	62	11	15	32	72	36
1949	118	32	2	0	9	59	16
Pre-1949	5,380	1,165	304	268	1,300	2,203	140

Note: These data are abstracted from a variety of state reports.

mildly or moderately retarded. After all, sterilization was usually performed upon persons thought capable of being discharged from the institution to the community.

Ironically, the less serious the retardation, the less likely that its cause
will be diagnosed and the less likely that it will be due to a Mendelian
disorder. But even among the more seriously retarded, Mendelian dis-

orders explain a relatively small fraction of cases. Consider a recent survey of the causes of major mental retardation (i.e., excluding the mildly retarded). Of 221 children with IQs less than 55, only 11 (4.9 percent) had a known Mendelian disorder. Of the rest, 58 had a chromosome disorder (most had Down syndrome), 24 had a known environmental cause, 23 had a recognized syndrome without a known inheritance pattern, and 13 were thought to suffer from problems related to labor and delivery. The rest were scattered among other nongenetic categories. The mental retardation of the largest group, 59 individuals, was considered to have no known cause.[26]

These findings are not much different from those uncovered in a survey of Fernald State School in Massachusetts in 1971. Of 1,378 residents, 1,077 had IQs below 50, and 301 had IQs of 50 or above. In the first group, no cause could be established for the retardation of 385 persons; in the second group, no cause could be found for that of 156 individuals. Although the survey did not tally Mendelian disorders, even a liberal estimate would indicate that fewer than 10 percent were so afflicted.[27]

Even as evidence mounted that most retardation did not have a Mendelian etiology, eugenicists persisted in asserting that there was a substantial likelihood that the offspring of persons born retarded would also be born retarded. Beginning in the early 1930s, a number of studies addressed this issue. One of the most important was a 1933 study in Birmingham, England, that analyzed the school performance of 345 children whose fathers or mothers had attended special schools for mental defectives (as the study called them). Only 25 of the 345 (7.5 percent) were themselves currently enrolled in special schools. Of the remaining 320 it was determined that 18 percent were "backward," but the vast majority were normal. Of this large group, there were 13 children for whom both parents were mentally defective. Only one of the 13 was considered to be retarded. This led J.B.S. Haldane, a leading population geneticist, to conclude that "it is never possible, from a knowledge of a person's parents to predict with certainty that he or she will be either a more adequate or a less adequate member of society than the majority."[28]

During the 1950s and 1960s, Sheldon Reed, a professor of human genetics at the University of Minnesota, carried out extensive research on the children born of unions in which one or both parents were retarded. The vast majority of the parents did not have a clear diagnosis, and Dr. Reed labeled them as polygenic or familial. He concluded that a couple's risk of bearing a retarded child was inversely proportional to parental intelligence and was higher if they already had an affected child. He estimated that in a marriage between a retarded and a nonretarded person, there was an 11 percent risk that they would produce a retarded child. Reed's findings certainly suggest that persons whose retardation is familial have a higher risk of bearing retarded children.[29] However, the study does not suggest that curtailing reproduction by retarded persons will significantly reduce the prevalence of this disorder in subsequent generations.

Perhaps the most interesting scientific advance in our understanding of the causes of mental retardation that is relevant to the eugenic thesis has been the delineation of Fragile X syndrome.[30] This familial disorder, in which women who are usually of normal intelligence carry a genetic defect that expresses itself as mental retardation in their sons, is roughly as common as Down syndrome. Although Fragile X does not really behave according to Mendelian laws (the details are beyond the scope of this book), by identifying carrier and affected individuals and curtailing their reproduction one still could sharply reduce the prevalence of the disorder. Nevertheless, the impact on the overall burden of mental retardation would be small, and the economic costs would be high. Further, it is unlikely that contemporary American society would or should tolerate programs to restrict the right to reproduce.

At the beginning of the 1990s, despite more than a century of interest, our understanding of the causes of mental retardation does not permit us to conclude that sterilization of retarded persons would significantly alter the prevalence of retardation in future generations. The non-Mendelian causes are simply much greater than the Mendelian contribution.

The Future of Involuntary Sterilization

Given the limits that the government has placed upon the use of federal funds to provide sterilization services to poor persons and the cautious manner in which state courts have handled petitions to sterilize retarded persons, the era of involuntary sterilization for eugenic reasons seems over. As we have seen, the more pressing problem currently is how to assert a retarded person's *right* to be sterilized.

The notion that selective sterilization could reap social benefits by reducing welfare costs does remain disturbingly attractive in some quarters. For example, during the 1960s a number of state legislatures considered bills that were designed to discourage the birth of illegitimate children. Mississippi and Louisiana adopted laws that made parenthood out of wedlock a crime punishable by thirty to ninety days in jail. In 1960 the Maryland Senate passed a bill that made it a felony to bear more than two illegitimate children, but the bill was rejected by the House of Delegates. Similarly, in 1967 an Ohio judge ruled that a woman with two illegitimate children had violated the state's child neglect law by failing to provide a "stable moral environment."[31] In several states, legislators considered offering child support subsidies only to those welfare mothers who agreed to be sterilized. In 1980 the chairman of the Board of Resources in Texas audaciously suggested that welfare recipients should have mandatory sterilizations.[32]

There have been no recent formal surveys of public opinion about involuntary sterilization, but it is at least possible that the popularity of tubal ligation and vasectomy as a family planning option will diminish concern about the threat posed to retarded persons by sterilization. The National Center for Health Statistics reported that by 1976 one-third of the nation's couples with wives of child-bearing age had chosen sterilization as a means of birth control.[33] Attitudes toward this surgery today are vastly different than they were sixty years ago, when people confused vasectomy with castration and the laparoscope had not yet been invented.

There have been some interesting unscientific opinion polls pertaining to involuntary sterilization. In 1981 a Texas legislator asked his Houston constituency whether they favored sterilization for women on welfare who had at least three children. They voted 3,533 to 2,604 in favor of keying welfare benefits to sterilization.[34] Lest one dismiss this as a quirk of Texas politics, consider the results of a telephone poll conducted by the *Boston Globe* in March 1982. The *Globe* asked: "Do you favor forced sterilizations for mentally ill persons?" Of 249 persons who called in with a response, 48 percent replied affirmatively.[35]

The suspicion that criminality lurks in the genes has a perennial popularity that extends into the scientific community. Dr. Sarnoff Mednick, a California psychologist, has persistently argued that a tendency toward criminality may be inherited.[36] The discovery in 1968 that persons with an extra Y chromosome were found more frequently than expected in mental-penal institutions intrigued a cohort of biologically oriented criminologists.[37] When interest in the XYY problem mushroomed, a federal agency, the Law Enforcement Assistance Administration, was quick to fund scientists to study "biological" criminality.

These anecdotes suggest that proposals to coerce people into submitting to sterilization will continue to arise. Welfare mothers, especially young women with several children, will probably continue to be a favorite target. But there are other circumstances in which sterilization may be proposed. It has become the policy of some employers to prevent fertile women from working in jobs that expose them to known or potential teratogens. In 1979 it was widely reported that five women who worked at the Willow Island, West Virginia, plant of American Cyanamid had undergone sterilization in order to keep jobs that exposed them to high levels of lead, a known teratogen. This led to an inspection by the Occupational Safety and Health Administration (OSHA), which concluded that the company had violated its general duty to provide a "place of employment free from recognized hazards that are causing or are likely to cause death or serious physical harm." The company challenged that citation, and the case was ultimately reviewed by the United States Court of Appeals. In an opinion written by Judge Robert Bork, the appellate court construed a key provision of the Occupational Safety and Health Act in a manner that placed the company's sterilization policy beyond its oversight, in effect validating American Cyanamid's approach to dealing with teratogen exposure.[38]

In the ensuing years, several major companies have disclosed that they have a policy of excluding fertile women from jobs they think expose workers to levels of a chemical that might be dangerous to a developing fetus. This has led to charges that the employers, who often lack solid data to support their policies, are using concern for "fetal rights" as a cover to discriminate against women.[39]

A few women have sued their employers, arguing that the choice between proof of infertility or exclusion from the workplace violates Title VII of the Civil Rights Act, a law that forbids job discrimination on the basis of gender. The issues posed are difficult, for they require weighing possible risks to unconceived children against real risks of employment discrimination. The courts have divided on how to handle these cases. In Ohio a federal district court ruled that a woman who was transferred away from exposure to vinyl chloride, but whose employer had not reduced her salary and who could show no evidence that the move would harm her career, did not have a Title VII claim. The court was sympathetic to the company's fear that it would be sued if the woman gave birth to a defective child.[40] In December 1982 the Circuit Court of Appeals ruled differently, holding that the Olin Corporation's policy of restricting access by fertile women to certain jobs because of a possible, but unknown, risk to a fetus could constitute a violation of Title VII.[41] In May 1990 the California Supreme Court upheld a lower court ruling that a woman could not be banned by her employer from a job that could harm a fetus she might be carrying.[42] The resolution of this problem does not belong to the courts. It requires a much more sophisticated understanding of the etiology of birth defects than we currently have. Nevertheless, I suspect that for now courts hearing Title VII claims will require employers to offer scientific evidence to support their job transfer policies. However, should there be a flurry of successful lawsuits brought by children with birth defects born to women who worked in toxic environments, appellate courts may show greater sympathy for preemptive acts by employers.

One could write an entire volume on the use of coercive sterilization in population control. While it is unlikely that such a policy would ever be launched in the United States, programs in India and China have already been deployed. In 1951 India became the first country to adopt a family planning program, but in the ensuing twenty years its population still grew from 356 million to 548 million. Faced with this explosion, the government began to support voluntary sterilization. But the population continued to grow, and in 1975 the government launched an ambitious plan to decrease the birth rate from 35 per 1,000 to 25 per 1,000 in less than ten years. The most dramatic expression of this policy was the adoption of a compulsory sterilization bill by the state of Maharashtra in 1976. The bill, which failed to become law when the president of India refused to sign it, provided that when a couple had three living children, the male partner had to undergo sterilization within 180 days of the birth of the third child. Exceptions were made for families in which all three children were of the same sex or if the youngest child was older than five. It provoked a storm of protest in India, and Prime Minister Desai quickly soft-pedaled government support of sterilization.[43]

Barely had the storm in India subsided when China's leaders announced that they were instituting a policy that favored the one-child family. Although the Chinese Communist regime had embraced a pronatalist policy when it came to power in 1949, by the late 1950s there was serious concern about the need to curb population growth. Between 1965 and the late 1970s, China managed to cut the crude birth rate from 37 per 1,000 to about 20 per 1,000. During this period, the main emphasis was on delaying marriage.

With its immense population base, even this dramatic reduction in fertility left China faced with a growth rate of more than one million people per month. Confronted with frightening predictions by its demographers, the Chinese leaders decided to aim for zero population growth by the year 2000. In 1979, China launched a "one-child pledge" program; and by 1980, the vigorous implementation of this policy had spurred a national debate. Rural communities and army leaders were among those who strongly opposed such a dramatic reduction, but the antigrowth forces prevailed. In 1981, the government introduced strong economic incentives to delay marriages and create a one-child limit per family. These incentives are enforced by intensive peer pressure. Compliant couples receive small supplementary monthly payments and food rations, free health care, schooling, preferences for housing and jobs, preferences for the child's higher education, and (for those who work directly for the state, mainly in urban areas) higher pensions. Couples who sign the pledge, but subsequently violate it by bearing a second child, must repay all one-child benefits they have received. Early reports from Sichuan, a province with 100 million people, claim that there was an astounding 72 percent reduction in the birth rate in the last few years.[44]

But China's birth control program has engendered much discontent. "People are going and knocking on doors every night and arguing with people who don't take the pledge," a correspondent quoted one foreign observer in Hebei Province as saying. Commune officials working in the campaign were warned that "you must not be afraid of being beaten." When asked about those who did not sign the pledge, one commune official responded simply: "Everybody is going to sign the pledge."[45] China's policy of one child per family has led a number of Chinese to seek political asylum in the United States. Immigration lawyers report that a number of their clients claim that they were forced to undergo sterilization. Representatives of the Chinese government have denied that forced sterilizations are carried out, but it appears that much pressure is placed on persons to submit voluntarily to the surgery.[46]

Given their aggressive approach to restricting population growth, it should come as no surprise that the Chinese routinely sterilize retarded persons. In 1989 the *New York Times* reported that one region of China had enacted a sterilization law not unlike those once so prevalent in the United States. During a single year the law, which targets married retarded persons, resulted in more than one thousand sterilizations. The *Times* noted that "the law has been hailed nationwide, and officials say that the national legislature and half a dozen provincial governments are thinking of adopting similar legislation."[47]

By alluding to the threat of involuntary sterilization in India and China, I do not mean to imply that the United States is at similar risk. In an era of limited resources and perennial debate over the cost of welfare programs, however, it is not fantastic to imagine campaigns to shape the child-bearing activities of certain groups of individuals. Individuals exposed to mutagenic or teratogenic agents, those incapable (whether for medical or economic reasons) of caring for their children, and persons at special risk for bearing infants with serious, incurable disorders are among the most obvious target groups. On at least one occasion, a couple with a child with cystic fibrosis (an incurable autosomal recessive disorder that affects the lungs and pancreas) were warned by staff at their health maintenance organization that coverage would not be extended to a second affected child. After complaints by the parents and the genetic counselors from whom the family sought prenatal diagnosis, the organization backed off.

The history of involuntary sterilization of institutionalized persons demonstrates that society has sometimes not hesitated to pursue what it perceived to be cost-saving measures at the expense of personal liberties. It is tempting to dismiss the stories of the Jukes and the Kallikaks and our society's reaction to them as quaint tales of a bygone era. The better course is to remember that in the name of science not so long ago, sixty thousand American citizens were subjected to eugenic sterilization. We must forever guard against the kind of flawed thinking that supported this activity.

Notes

Chapter 1: The Heritability of Degeneracy

1. A. E. Sturtevant, "The early Mendelians," *Proc. Amer. Phil. Soc.*, 1965, 109 (no. 4): 199-204.
2. F. Galton, *Hereditary Genius: An Inquiry into Its Laws and Consequences* (London: Macmillan, 1869), p. 14.
3. F. Galton, *English Men of Science: Their Nature and Nurture* (London: Macmillan, 1874).
4. D. W. Forrest, *Francis Galton: The Life and Work of a Victorian Genius* (New York: Taplinger, 1974), p. 122.
5. F. Galton, *Inquiries into Human Faculty and Its Development* (London: Macmillan, 1883).
6. Forrest, *Francis Galton*, p. 260.
7. A. Weismann, *The Germ-Plasm: A Theory of Heredity* (London: Walter Scott, 1893).
8. E. Haeckel, *The Evolution of Man* (New York: Appleton, 1896).
9. R. Hofstadter, *Social Darwinism in American Thought* (Boston: Beacon Press, 1965), p. 33.
10. H. Spencer, *Social Statistics* (London: John Chapman, 1851), p 44.
11. J. C. Greene, "Some early speculations on the origin of human races," *Amer. Anthropol.*, 1954, 56: 31-41.
12. W. Stanton, *The Leopard's Spots: Scientific Attitudes toward Race in America, 1815-1859* (Chicago: University of Chicago Press, 1960), pp. 1-14.
13. S. G. Morton, *Crania Americana* (Philadelphia: John Pennington, 1839).
14. S. J. Gould, *The Mismeasure of Man* (New York: Norton, 1981), p. 171.
15. E. Jarvis, "Statistics of insanity in the United States," *Boston Med. Surg. J.*, 1842, 27: 116-21, 281-82.
16. A. Deutsch, "The first U.S. census of the insane (1840), and its use as pro-slavery propaganda," *Bull. Hist. Med.*, 1944, 5: 469-82.
17. J. C. Nott, "The mulatto a hybrid—probable extermination of the two races if the whites and blacks are allowed to intermarry," *Am. J. Med. Sci.*, 1843, 6: 252-56.
18. Stanton, *Leopard's Spots*, p. 175.
19. G. Lombroso-Ferrero, *Lombroso's Criminal Man* (reprint, Montclair, New Jersey: Patterson Smith, 1972), p. vii.
20. Ibid., pp. xxiv-xxv.
21. H. M. Boies, *Prisoners and Paupers* (New York: Putnam, 1893), pp. 267-68.

22. Ibid., pp. 269-70.
23. A. H. Estabrook, *The Jukes in 1915* (Washington, D.C.: Carnegie Institute, 1916), pp. v-vi.
24. R. L. Dugdale, *The Jukes: A Study in Crime, Pauperism, and Heredity*, 4th ed. (New York: Putnam, 1910), p. 7.
25. Ibid., pp. 26-27.
26. R. L. Dugdale, "Hereditary pauperism as illustrated in the Juke family" (Paper read at the American Social Science Association meetings, Saratoga, New York. This paper is cited in *The Jukes in 1915*, p. 1).

Chapter 2: The Cost of Degeneracy

1. R. C. Scheerenberger, *A History of Mental Retardation* (Baltimore: Brookes, 1983), pp. 109-36.
2. "Status of the Work before the People and the Legislatures," in *The Proceedings of the Association of Medical Officers of American Institutions for Idiotic and Feeble-Minded Persons* (hereafter *Proc. AMO*) (Philadelphia: Lippincott, 1878), p. 96.
3. Ibid., pp. 103-6.
4. "Status of the Work," in *Proc. AMO* (Philadelphia: Lippincott, 1880), pp. 163-66.
5. "Status of the Work," in *Proc. AMO* (Philadelphia: Lippincott, 1885), p. 361.
6. "Status of the Work," in *Proc. AMO* (Philadelphia: Lippincott, 1888), pp. 77-78.
7. R. A. Mott, "Welcoming Remarks," in *Proc. AMO* (Philadelphia: Lippincott, 1890), pp. 117-22.
8. A. W. Wilmarth, "Presidential Address," in *Proc. AMO* (Philadelphia: Lippincott, 1895), p. 607.
9. Dugdale, *The Jukes*, p. 167.
10. I. Kerlin, "Report to the Eleventh National Conference of Charities and Reforms," in *Proc. AMO* (1885), p. 404.
11. I. Kerlin, "Report of Standing Committee on Provision for Idiots," in *Proc. AMO* (Philadelphia: Lippincott, 1886), pp. 506-7.
12. O. McCulloch, "The Tribe of Ishmael: A Study in Social Degradation," in *Proc. Fifteenth Nat. Conf. Char. Corrections* (Buffalo, N.Y., 1888).
13. Boies, *Prisoners and Paupers*, p. 10.
14. F. W. Robertson, "Sterilization for the criminal unfit," *Amer. Med.*, 1910, 5: 349-61.
15. Dugdale, *The Jukes*, p. 160.
16. C. E. Rosenberg, "Charles Benedict Davenport and the beginning of human genetics," *Bull. Hist. Med.*, 1961, 35: 266-76.
17. C. B. Davenport, "Heredity of some human physical characteristics," *Proc. Soc. Exp. Biol. Med.*, 1908, 5: 101-2.
18. G. E. Allen, "The Role of Experts in Scientific Controversy," in *Scientific Controversies: Case Studies in the Resolution and Closure of Disputes in Science and Technology*, ed. H. T. Engelhardt, Jr., and A. L. Caplan (Cambridge: Cambridge University Press, 1987), p. 183.
19. F. Danielson and C. Davenport, *The Hill Folk: Report on a Rural Community*

of Hereditary Defectives (Cold Spring Harbor, New York: Eugenics Record Office, 1912), pp. 11-12.

20. A. Estabrook and C. Davenport, *The Nam Family: A Study in Cacogenics* (Cold Spring Harbor, New York: Eugenics Record Office, 1912), p. 1.
21. Estabrook, *Jukes in 1915,* p. 1.
22. H. H. Goddard, *The Kallikak Family* (New York: Macmillan, 1912).
23. The biographical material on Goddard is based largely on an interview with Dr. M. S. Crissey at her home in Flint, Michigan, in 1982. She did graduate work with Dr. Goddard.
24. H. H. Goddard, *Heredity of Feeblemindedness,* Bulletin no. 1 (Cold Spring Harbor, New York: Eugenics Record Office, 1910).
25. H. H. Goddard, *Feeble-mindedness: Its Causes and Consequences* (New York: Macmillan, 1914).
26. M. S. Crissey, "Ghosts of the Jersey pines," Paper delivered at the Annual Meeting of the American Psychological Association, New York, Sept. 4, 1979.
27. Goddard, *Kallikak Family,* p. 50.
28. Gould, *Mismeasure of Man,* p. 171.
29. J. Higham, *Strangers in the Land* (New York: Atheneum, 1965), p. 72.
30. Ibid., p. 104.
31. R. L. Garis, *Immigration Restriction* (New York: Macmillan, 1927), pp. 239-49.
32. Ibid., pp. 89-102.
33. Ibid., p. 112.
34. K. M. Ludmerer, *Genetics and American Society* (Baltimore: Johns Hopkins Press, 1972).
35. W. Wadlington, "The Loving case: Virginia's antimiscegenation statute in historical perspective," *Virg. Law Rev.,* 1966, 52: 1189-1223.
36. J. G. Mencke, *Mulattoes and Race Mixture: American Attitudes and Images, 1865-1918* (Ann Arbor: UMI Research Press, 1959), p. C39.
37. "Intermarriage with negroes—a survey of the states," *Yale Law J.,* 1927, 36: 858-66, 862.
38. H. M. Applebaum, "Miscegenation statutes: a constitutional and social problem," *Georgetown Law J.,* 1964, 53: 49-91.
39. "Status of the Work," in *Proc. AMU* (Philadelphia: Lippincott, 1886), p. 350.
40. Mott, "Welcoming Remarks," p. 117.
41. Wilmarth, "Presidential Address," p. 607.
42. "Report of the Standing Committee on the Criminal Law," in *Proc. Ann. Cong. Nat. Prison Assoc. U.S.* (Pittsburgh: NPA Press, 1897), p. 152.
43. C. B. Davenport, *State Laws Limiting Marriage Selection* (Cold Spring Harbor, New York: Eugenics Record Office, 1913).
44. C. B. Davenport, *Huntington's Chorea in Relation to Heredity and Eugenics,* Bulletin no. 17 (Cold Spring Harbor, New York: Eugenics Record Office, 1916).
45. Davenport, *State Laws Limiting Marriage Selection,* p. 44.
46. *Gould v. Gould,* 78 Conn. 242, 61 Atl. 604 (1905).
47. G. L. Cannon and A. J. Rosanoff, "Preliminary report of a study of heredity in insanity in the light of the Mendelian laws," *J. Nerv. Ment. Dis.,* 1911, 38 (no. 5): 272-79.

48. F. E. Daniel, "Emasculation for criminal assaults and for incest," *Tex. Med. J.*, 1907, 22: 347.
49. P. I. Nixon, "A pioneer Texas emasculator: a chapter from the life of Dr. Gideon Lincecum," *Tex. Med. Hist.*, May 1940, 34-48.
50. F. E. Daniel, "Emasculation of masturbators—is it justifiable?" *Tex. Med. J.*, 1894, 10: 239-44.

Chapter 3: The Surgical Solution

1. A. J. Ochsner, "Surgical treatment of habitual criminals," *JAMA*, 1899, 53: 867-68.
2. J. E. Mears, "Asexualization as a remedial measure in the relief of certain forms of mental, moral, and physical degeneration," *Boston Med. Surg. J.*, 1909, 161: 584-86.
3. *Dictionary of American Biography*, vol. 13 (1934), s.v. "Oschner, Albert John."
4. H. C. Sharp, "The severing of the vasa deferentia and its relation to the neuropsychopathic constitution," *N.Y. Med. J.*, 1902, 411-14.
5. Ibid., p. 411.
6. R. C. Ellinwood, "Vasectomy," *Cal. St. Med. J.*, 1904, 2: 60-62.
7. S. D. Risley, "Is asexualization ever justifiable in the case of imbecile children?" *J. Psycho-Asthenics*, 1905, 9: 92-98.
8. H. H. Laughlin, *Eugenical Sterilization in the United States* (Chicago: Chicago Psychopathic Laboratory, 1922).
9. H. C. Sharp, "Rendering Sterile of Confirmed Criminals and Mental Defectives," *Proc. Ann. Cong. Nat. Prison Assoc. U.S.* (Pittsburgh: NPA Press, 1907), pp. 177-85.
10. M. Madlener, "Uber sterilisierende operationen an den tuben," *Zentralbl. F. Gynak.*, 1919, 43: 380-84.
11. American Urological Association, *History of Urology*, ed. E. G. Ballenger et al. (Baltimore: Williams & Wilkins, 1954), pp. 50-51.
12. W. T. Belfield, "Race suicide for social parasites," *JAMA*, 1908, 50: 55-56.
13. Mears, "Asexualization as a remedial measure."
14. H. C. Sharp, "Vasectomy as a means of preventing procreation of defectives," *JAMA*, 1909, 53: 1897-1902.
15. Ibid., p. 1902.
16. C. B. Davenport and D. F. Weeks, *A First Study of Inheritance in Epilepsy* (Cold Spring Harbor, New York: Eugenics Record Office, 1911).
17. C. V. Carrington, "Sterilization of habitual criminals," *Virg. Med. Semi-Mo.*, 1909, 36: 421-22.
18. P. Popenoe, "The progress of eugenic sterilization," *J. Heredity*, 1933, 28: 19-25.
19. L. F. Barker, "The importance of the eugenic movement and its relation to social hygiene," *JAMA*, 1910, 54: 2017-22.
20. G. F. Lydston, "Sex mutilations in social therapeutics," *N.Y. Med. J.*, 1912, 95: 677-85.
21. *Dictionary of American Biography*, vol. 11 (1933), s.v. "Lydston, George Frank."
22. G. F. Lydston, *Diseases of Society* (Philadelphia: Lippincott, 1906), p. 564.
23. Ibid.

24. F. E. Daniel, "Castration of sexual perverts," *Tex. Med. J.,* 1894, 12: 255.
25. F. E. Daniel, "Sterilization bill rejected," *Tex. Med. J.,* 1907, 23: 42-44.
26. F. E. Daniel, "Sterilization of male insane," *Tex. Med. J.,* 1909, 25: 110-12.
27. Popenoe, "Progress of eugenic sterilization," p. 23.
28. B. Owens-Adair, "Human sterilization," Undated pamphlet, Sterling Memorial Library, Yale University, New Haven, Connecticut.
29. J. H. Landman, *Human Sterilization* (New York: Macmillan, 1932).

Chapter 4: Sterilization Laws

1. Rhode Island State Library Legislative Reference Bureau, "Sterilization of the unfit," Undated pamphlet, Connecticut State Library, Hartford.
2. Laughlin, *Eugenical Sterilization in the United States.*
3. W. W. Foster, "Hereditary criminality and its certain cure," *Pearson's Magazine,* Nov. 1909, pp. 565-72.
4. "The science of breeding better men," *Scientific American,* 1911, 104: 562.
5. See the Davenport-Harriman Letters in the Charles Benedict Davenport Papers (hereafter Davenport Papers), Laughlin folder 2, American Philosophical Society Library, Philadelphia.
6. C. B. Davenport (C.B.D.) to H. H. Laughlin (H.H.L.), Nov. 28, 1911, Davenport Papers, Laughlin folder 2.
7. *Proceedings of the Third Race Betterment Conference* (Battle Creek, Michigan: Race Betterment Foundation, 1928).
8. T. R. Roosevelt, "Twisted eugenics," *Outlook,* 1904, 106: 30-34.
9. M. Grant, *The Passing of the Great Race* (New York: Scribner, 1916).
10. F. Boas, *Changes in Bodily Form of Descendants of Immigrants,* Report by the Immigration Commission to the Committee on Immigration of the 61st Congress (Washington, D.C.: GPO, 1910).
11. A. Johnson, "Race improvement by control of defectives (negative eugenics)," *Ann. Am. Acad. Penal Soc. Sci.,* 1910, 34: 22-29.
12. F. Boas, "Eugenics," *Scientific Monthly,* 1916, 3: 471-78.
13. L. Ward, "Eugenics, euthenics, and endemics," *Am J. Soc.,* 1913, 18: 737-54.
14. Editorial, *New York Times,* "Race homicide," n.d., quoted in *Medico-Legal J.,* 1910, 27: 140.
15. Rhode Island State Library Legislative Reference Bureau, "Sterilization of the unfit," pp. 18-19.
16. Laughlin, *Eugenical Sterilization in the United States,* pp. 1-96.
17. Ibid., p. 19.
18. Ibid., p. 9.
19. Ibid., p. 42.
20. Ibid., p. 85.
21. Ibid., p. 86.
22. Ibid., p. 71.
23. Ibid., p. 72.
24. Ibid., p. 73.
25. *State v. Feilen,* 70 Wash. 65, 126 P. 75 (1912).
26. *Mickle v. Henrichs,* 262 F. 687 (1918).
27. *Smith v. Board of Examiners of Feeble-Minded,* 88 Atl. 963 (1918).
28. *Davis v. Berry,* 216 F. 413 (1914).

29. *In re Thomson,* 103 Misc. Rep. 23, 169 N.Y.S. 638 (1918).
30. Laughlin, *Eugenical Sterilization in the United States,* pp. 22-24.
31. E. R. Spaulding and W. Healy, "Inheritance as a Factor in Criminality," in *The Physical Bases of Crime* (Easton, Pennsylvania: American Academy of Medicine Press, 1914), pp. 19-42.

Chapter 5: Harry H. Laughlin: Champion of Sterilization

1. *Dictionary of American Biography,* suppl. 3 (1941-45), s.v. "Laughlin, Harry Hamilton."
2. H.H.L. to C.B.D., Feb. 25, 1907, Davenport Papers, Laughlin folder 1.
3. H.H.L. to C.B.D., Mar. 30, 1908, Davenport Papers, Laughlin folder 1.
4. C.B.D. to H.H.L., Dec. 24, 1908, Davenport Papers, Laughlin folder 1.
5. C.B.D. to M. W. Harriman, Davenport Papers, Laughlin folder 1.
6. F. J. Hassencahl, "Harry H. Laughlin, Expert Eugenics Agent for the House Committee on Immigration and Naturalization, 1921 to 1931" (Ph.D. diss., Case Western Reserve University, 1970; Ann Arbor: Univ. Microfilms, 50).
7. C. B. Davenport, "Report of Committee on Eugenics (Report of the meeting held in Omaha, December 8-10, 1910, and for the year ending December 31, 1909)," *Amer. Breeders Assoc.,* 1911, 6: 92-94.
8. Hassencahl, "Laughlin," pp. 95-97.
9. H. H. Laughlin, *The Scope of the Committee's Work,* Bulletin no. 10A (Cold Spring Harbor, New York: Eugenics Record Office, 1914), pp. 12-14.
10. H. H. Laughlin, *The Legal, Legislative, and Administrative Aspects of Sterilization,* Bulletin no. 10B (Cold Spring Harbor, New York: Eugenics Record Office, 1914).
11. H. H. Laughlin, "Calculations on the Working Out of a Proposed Program of Sterilization," in *Proc. Nat. Conf. Race Betterment,* Jan. 8-12, 1914 (Battle Creek, Michigan: Race Betterment Foundation, 1914), pp. 478-92.
12. Hassencahl, "Laughlin," p. 62.
13. H. H. Laughlin, "The dynamics of cell division," *Proc. Soc. Exp. Biol. Med.,* 1918, 15 (no. 8): 32-44.
14. H.H.L. to C.B.D., Mar. 11, 1916, Davenport Papers, Laughlin folder 3.
15. H. H. Laughlin, "Nativity of Institutional Inmates," in *Eugenics in Race and State,* vol. 2, Scientific Papers of the Second International Congress of Eugenics, 1921 (Baltimore: Williams & Wilkins, 1923), pp. 402-6.
16. C. B. Davenport, "Eugenics Record Office," in *Carnegie Institute Yearbook 18* (Washington, D.C.: Carnegie Institute, 1919), p. 149.
17. K. B. Davis to R. D. Fosdick, Apr. 14, 1921, Davenport Papers, Laughlin folder 7.
18. See Chapter 3, note 7, for full citation.
19. H. H. Laughlin, "Biological Aspects of Immigration," in *Hearings before the Committee on Immigration and Naturalization, House of Representatives,* 66th Cong., 2d sess. (Washington, D.C.: GPO, 1921).
20. Hassencahl, "Laughlin," p. 179.
21. H. H. Laughlin, "Analysis of America's Modern Melting Pot," in *Hearings before the House Committee on Immigration and Naturalization, House of Representatives,* 67th Cong., 3d sess. (Washington, D.C.: GPO, 1922).

22. B. Lasker to H. Jennings, Nov. 24, 1923, quoted in Ludmerer, *Genetics and American Society,* p. 103.
23. Letter from R. Pearl to H. Jennings, Nov. 24, 1923, quoted in ibid., p. 113.
24. Garis, *Immigration Restriction,* pp. 240-51.
25. Hassencahl, "Laughlin," p. 190.
26. H. H. Laughlin, "Europe as an Emigrant Exporting Continent and the United States as an Immigrant Receiving Nation," in *Hearings before the House Committee on Immigration and Naturalization,* 68th Cong., 1st sess. (Washington, D.C.: GPO, 1924).
27. H. H. Laughlin, *Eugenical Sterilization: 1926* (New Haven: American Eugenics Society, 1926).
28. H. H. Laughlin, "Eugenical sterilization of the feeble-minded," *J. Psycho-Asthenics,* 1926, 31: 210-18.
29. "Harvard declines a legacy to found a eugenics course," *New York Times,* May 7, 1927, clipping in Harry Hamilton Laughlin Archives, Pickler Memorial Library, Northeast Missouri State University, Kirksville, Missouri (hereafter, Laughlin Archives).
30. R. J. Cynkar, "*Buck v. Bell:* 'Felt Necessities' v. 'Fundamental Values?'" *Colum. Law Rev.,* 1981, 81: 1418-61.
31. Ibid., pp. 1438-39.
32. *Buck v. Bell,* 274 U.S. 200 (1927).
33. Hassencahl, "Laughlin," p. 321.
34. C.B.D. to C. C. Tegethoff, Nov. 7, 1914, Davenport Papers, Eugenics Record Office folder.
35. C.B.D. to H.H.L., Apr. 16, 1928, Davenport Papers, Laughlin folder 21.
36. Memorandum for Dr. Laughlin from C.B.D., Apr. 19, 1929, Davenport Papers, Laughlin folder 22.
37. "Relaxing quotas for exiles fought," *New York Times,* May 4, 1934, clipping in Laughlin Archives.
38. "A long-wanted textbook," *Saturday Evening Post,* Aug. 4, 1934, clipping in Laughlin Archives.
39. L. C. Dunn to J. C. Merriam, July 3, 1935, Davenport Papers, Laughlin folder 32.
40. J. C. Merriam to H. H. Laughlin, Dec. 31, 1938, Davenport Papers, Laughlin folder 37.
41. Personal communication from Dr. Sheldon Reed, University of Minnesota, Dec. 14, 1982.

Chapter 6: The Resurgence of Eugenics

1. Laughlin, *Eugenical Sterilization in the United States,* pp. 1-50.
2. Second International Congress of Eugenics, *Eugenics, Genetics, and the Family,* ed. Committee on Publication (C. B. Davenport, H. F. Osborn, C. Wissler, and H. H. Laughlin), vol. 1 (Baltimore: Williams & Wilkins, 1923).
3. Second International Congress of Eugenics, *Eugenics in Race and State,* vol. 2 (Baltimore: Williams & Wilkins, 1923).
4. Wadlington, "The Loving case," pp. 1189-1223.
5. Mencke, *Mulattoes and Race Mixture,* p. 39.

6. Virginia Acts of Assembly, 1924, chap. 371.
7. H. M. Applebaum, "Miscegenation statutes: a constitutional and social problem," *Georgetown Law J.,* 1964, 53: 49-91.
8. L. Thompson and W. S. Downs, eds., *Who's Who in American Medicine 1925* (New York: Macmillan, 1925).
9. H.H.L. to W. A. Plecker, Feb. 23, 1928, Laughlin Archives.
10. W.A.P. to H.H.L., Feb. 25, 1928, Laughlin Archives.
11. W.A.P. to H.H.L., Nov. 28, 1928, Laughlin Archives.
12. W.A.P. to Stewart, May 24, 1929, Laughlin Archives.
13. W.A.P. to H.H.L., May 24, 1929, Laughlin Archives.
14. W.A.P. to H.H.L., Mar. 19, 1930, Laughlin Archives.
15. W.A.P. to H.H.L., June 18, 1931, Laughlin Archives.
16. C. B. Davenport, *Heredity of Skin Color in Negro-White Crosses* (Washington, D.C.: Carnegie Institute, 1913), p. 29.
17. M. Parmelee, *Criminology* (New York: Macmillan, 1918), pp. 128-31.
18. E. H. Sutherland, *Criminology* (Philadelphia: Lippincott, 1924), pp. 621-22.
19. F. Strother, "The cause of crime: defective brain," *World's Work,* 1924, 48: 275-81.
20. "Hickson back ready to test gunmen's minds," *Chicago Daily Tribune,* p. 12, Undated clipping in Laughlin Archives.
21. F. Strother, "The cure for crime," *World's Work,* 1924, 48: 389-95.
22. F. Strother, "How human traits are inherited," *World's Work,* 1925, 49: 281-86.
23. H. Olson, "Crime and Heredity," in *Research Studies of Crime* (Chicago: Municipal Court, 1926), pp. 9-61.
24. Memorandum from H.H.L. to the Eugenics Society of the United States of America on the matter of the proposed state aid in New York for local classes for the feebleminded, Mar. 23, 1923, Laughlin Archives.
25. L. F. Whitney, *The Basis of Breeding* (New Haven: Fowler, 1928).
26. E. Huntington to H. F. Perkins, Oct. 19, 1936, Ellsworth Huntington Archives, Unnumbered folder, Manuscripts and Archives, Yale University Library, New Haven, Connecticut (hereafter Huntington Archives).
27. I. Fisher, Memorandum to E. Huntington, Undated, Huntington Archives, folder 307.
28. E. P. Hamilton (J. Wiley & Sons) to E. Huntington, Sept. 8, 1936, Huntington Archives, folder 319.
29. Program of the American Eugenics Society (draft), sec. 9, Dec. 22, 1937, Huntington Archives, folder 347.
30. C. B. Davenport to E. Huntington, Apr. 3, 1937, Huntington Archives, folder 284.
31. F. Osborn to E. Huntington, May 10, 1938, Irving Fisher Archives, Manuscripts and Archives, Yale University Library, New Haven, Connecticut.
32. S. J. Holmes to F. Osborn, May 19, 1938, Huntington Archives, Unnumbered folder.
33. W. Kaempffert to F. Osborn, Aug. 31, 1939, Huntington Archives, Unnumbered folder.
34. *Pasadena Community Book* (1943), s.v. "Ezra Seymour Gosney."
35. E.S.G. to H.H.L., Jan. 26, 1926, Laughlin Archives.
36. E.S.G to H.H.L., Feb. 13, 1926, Laughlin Archives.

37. H.H.L. to E.S.G., Mar. 3, 1926, Laughlin Archives.
38. E.S.G. to H.H.L., Mar. 10, 1926, Laughlin Archives.
39. P. Popenoe, "Sterilization and Criminality," in *Proc. Fifty-First Ann. Meet. Am. Bar Assoc.* (Chicago: ABA Press, 1928), pp. 575-81.
40. E. S. Gosney and P. Popenoe, *Sterilization for Human Betterment* (New York: Macmillan, 1929).
41. Human Betterment Foundation, "Annual report for the year 1935," Feb. 6, 1936, Association for Voluntary Sterilization Records, Social Welfare History Archives, University of Minnesota, Minneapolis, Minnesota (hereafter AVS Archives).
42. D. H. Brush, "The Brush Foundation," *Eugenics,* 1929, 2 (no. 2): 17-19.
43. B. Shepard, "Purpose of the Brush Foundation," in *Race Betterment,* Brush Foundation Pub. no. 4 (Dayton, Ohio: Ohio Race Betterment Association, 1929), pp. 11-15.
44. W. S. Pritchard, "The Principle of Population," in *Race Betterment,* Brush Foundation Pub. no. 4 (Dayton, Ohio: Ohio Race Betterment Association, 1929), pp. 17-20.
45. R. Miles to V. Wing, secretary, Ohio Race Betterment Association, Sept. 12, 1930, Laughlin Archives.
46. H.H.L. to J. Fisher, Jan. 8, 1931, Laughlin Archives.
47. "Harvard declines a legacy to found a eugenics course," *New York Times,* May 7, 1927, Clipping in Laughlin Archives.
48. *Estate of J. Ewing Mears, Deceased,* Pennsylvania Sup. Ct. Case no. 124, January Term, 1930, Laughlin Archives.
49. R. V. Patterson to H. H. Laughlin, Nov. 24, 1931, Laughlin Archives.
50. E. Huntington to F. Osborn, Dec. 19, 1938, E. Huntington Archives.
51. M. Hillel and C. Henry, *Of Pure Blood* (New York: McGraw-Hill, 1976).
52. F. Osborn to E. Huntington, May 22, 1939, Huntington Archives, folder 349.
53. Laughlin, *The Legal Status of Eugenical Sterilization,* p. 49.
54. Rhode Island State Library Legislative Reference Bureau, "Sterilization of Degenerates," 1925, Pamphlet collection, Connecticut State Library, Hartford.
55. Ibid., p. 3.
56. Ibid., p. 4.
57. Ibid., p. 6.
58. *Smith v. Probate,* 231 Mich. 409 (1925).
59. Laughlin, *Eugenical Sterilization,* p. 148.
60. Cynkar, *Buck v. Bell,* pp. 1418-61.
61. *Buck v. Bell,* 143 Va. 310 (1925).
62. Cynkar, *Buck v. Bell,* p. 1439.
63. *Buck v. Bell,* 274 U.S. 200 (1927), p. 205.
64. Cynkar, *Buck v. Bell,* p. 1450.

Chapter 7: Sterilization Data

1. M. S. Edwards, "Legislative trends in 1931," *J. Soc. Hygiene,* 1931, 17: 402.
2. R. Johnson, "Legislation," *Eugenics,* 1931, 4 (no. 1): 28.
3. "Eugenical sterilization at the meeting of the A.M.A," *Eugenical News,* 1928, 13: 115.

4. "Notes and news," *Eugenical News,* 1929, 14: 136.
5. H. M. Watkins, "Selective sterilization," *J. Psycho-Asthenics,* 1930, 35: 51-67.
6. M. W. Barr and E. A. Whitney, "Preventive medicine and mental deficiency," *N.E.J. Med.,* 1930, 203: 872-76.
7. E. A. Whitney and M. M. Shick, "Some results of selective sterilization," *J. Psycho-Asthenics,* 1931, 36: 330-38.
8. E. B. Swanson, "A biographical sketch of Charles Fremont Dight, M.D.," in *Bulletin No. 1* (Minneapolis: Dight Institute, 1943), pp. 14-15.
9. F. Kuhlman to C. F. Dight, Feb. 14, 1927, Charles Fremont Dight Papers, box 10, Minnesota Historical Society, St. Paul, Minnesota.
10. D. G. Taylor to R.P.C. Wilson, Nov. 19, 1933, Robert P. C. Wilson Papers, Western Historical Manuscript Collection, University of Missouri, Columbia, Missouri.
11. R.P.C. Wilson to F. A. Carmichael, Jan. 12, 1937, Robert P. C. Wilson Papers.
12. R. H. Johnson, "Legislation," *Eugenics,* 1929, 2 (no. 6): 29.
13. R. H. Johnson, "Legislation," *Eugenics,* 1931, 4 (no. 1): 28.
14. Watkins, "Selective sterilization," pp. 51-67.
15. L. P. Harshman, "Medical and legal aspects of sterilization in Indiana," *J. Psycho-Asthenics,* 1935, 40: 58-68.
16. Ibid.
17. A. L. Develin to E.S.G., Jan. 9, 1933, AVS Archives.
18. C. Denham to E.S.G., Feb. 17, 1933, AVS Archives.
19. W. D. Partlow to E.S.G., Mar. 26, 1934, AVS Archives.
20. W. F. Dunham to E.S.G., Jan. 9, 1935, AVS Archives.
21. F. O. Willhite to E.S.G., Mar. 21, 1934, AVS Archives.
22. R. E. Brown to E.S.G., Mar. 24, 1934, AVS Archives.
23. Dept. of Public Welfare, Boise, Idaho, to E.S.G., Jan. 9, 1935, AVS Archives.
24. Utah State Training School, American Fork, Utah, to H.B.F., reporting on 1939, Undated, AVS Archives.
25. S. B. Folsom to E.S.G., Feb. 21, 1936, AVS Archives.
26. F. L. McAvinchey to P. Popenoe, June 24, 1936, AVS Archives.
27. T. C. Dale to J. G. Crick, Feb. 5, 1941, AVS Archives.
28. State Board of Control of Wisconsin, *Thirteenth Biennial Report: Period Ending June 30, 1916* (Madison: Democratic Printing, 1916), p. 6.
29. State Board of Control of Wisconsin, *Twenty-first Biennial Report: Period Ending June 30, 1932* (Madison: Democratic Printing, 1932), p. 26.
30. E. J. Engberg, "The sterilization of mental defectives in Minnesota," *J. Psycho-Asthenics,* 1939, 44: 167-72.
31. G. B. Arnold, "A brief review of the first thousand patients eugenically sterilized at the state colony for epileptics and feeble-minded," *J. Psycho-Asthenics,* 1938, 43: 56-83.
32. B. W. Baker, "Parole and sterilization," *Training School Bulletin,* 1939, 35: 177-87.
33. Gosney and Popenoe, *Sterilization for Human Betterment,* p. 132.
34. J. H. Craft, "The effects of sterilization," *J. Heredity,* 1936, 27: 379-87.
35. M. Woodside, *Sterilization in North Carolina* (Chapel Hill: Univ. North Carolina Press, 1950).
36. E. J. Engberg, "The sterilization of mental defectives in Minnesota," *J. Psycho-Asthenics,* 1939, 44: 167-72.

37. State Board of Control of Wisconsin, *Nineteenth Biennial Report: Period Ending June 30, 1928* (Madison: Democratic Printing, 1928), p. 28.
38. State Board of Control of Minnesota, *Thirteenth Biennial Report: Period Ending June 30, 1926* (Stillwater: State Prison Printing Dept., 1926), pp. 98-99.
39. State Board of Control of Minnesota, *Fourteenth Biennial Report: Period Ending June 30, 1928* (Stillwater: State Prison Printing Dept., 1928), p. 42.
40. Craft, "Effects of sterilization," p. 82.
41. Arnold, "Brief review," p. 69.
42. Baker, "Parole and sterilization," p. 183.
43. H. Maier, "On practical experience of sterilization in Switzerland," *Eugenics Rev.*, 1934, 26: 19-25.
44. G. R. Searle, *Eugenics and Politics in Britain, 1900-1914* (Leyden: Noordhoff International, 1976), p. 93.
45. Ibid., p. 242.
46. *Report of the Departmental Committee on Sterilization* (London: HMSO, 1934).
47. H. Herd, "Sterilization of the mentally defective," *Lancet*, Sept. 30, 1933, pp. 783-86.
48. F. D. Turner, "Mental deficiency and sterilization," *Med. Officer*, 1933, 50: 121-23.
49. D. Gibson, "Involuntary sterilization of the mentally retarded: a western Canadian phenomenon," *Can. Psychiatr. Assoc. J.*, 1974, 19: 59-63.
50. F. Lenz, "Eugenics in Germany," *J. Heredity*, 1924, 15: 223-31.
51. Ibid.
52. Ibid.
53. Quoted in P. Popenoe, "The German sterilization law," *J. Heredity*, 1935, 26: 257-60.
54. Ibid.
55. M. Kopp, "The German sterilization program," Undated typescript, AVS Archives.
56. H. H. Laughlin to H. Olson, Feb. 11, 1927, Laughlin Archives.
57. Hassencahl, "Laughlin," p. 350.
58. Popenoe, "German sterilization law," p. 258.
59. Kopp, "German sterilization program," p. 8.
60. R. Cook, "A year of German sterilization," *J. Heredity*, 1935, 26: 485-89.
61. W. C. Whiteside, "Leber's hereditary optic neuritis through six generations: a sterilization problem," *Can. Med. Assoc. J.*, 1939, 39: 347-48.
62. R. Cook, "Errors in German sterilization totals," *J. Heredity*, 1936, 27: 26.
63. For an excellent discussion of the influence of eugenics in Germany, see R. Proctor, *Racial Hygiene* (Cambridge: Harvard University Press, 1988).
64. "Summary of Swedish laws on sterilization, abortion, and castration," Typescript, May 1951, AVS Archives.
65. H. Von Hofsten, "Steriliseringar i Sverige, 1935-39," *Nordisk Med.*, 1940, 7 (no. 34): 1417-30, English summary, AVS Archives.
66. "Germans made sterile by Nazis seek pensions," *New York Herald Tribune*, Jan. 14, 1951.
67. Hillel and Henry, *Of Pure Blood*, p. 192.
68. "German Sterilization by Death Sentence," Summary of SHAEF Intelligence investigation, AVS Archives.

Chapter 8: Critics

1. Rosenberg, "Davenport and the beginning of human genetics."
2. M. Haller, *Eugenics: Hereditarian Attitudes in American Thought* (New Brunswick, New Jersey: Rutgers Univ. Press, 1963), p. 167.
3. R. C. Punnett, "Eliminating feeblemindedness," *J. Heredity*, 1917, 8: 464-65.
4. Ludmerer, *Genetics and American Society*, pp. 179-89.
5. H. S. Jennings, "Undesirable aliens," *Survey*, Dec. 15, 1923, pp. 309-12, 364.
6. H. S. Jennings, "Proportions of defectives from the Northwest and from the Southwest of Europe," *Science*, 1924, 59: 256-57.
7. H. S. Jennings, *The Biological Basis of Human Nature* (New York: Norton, 1930), p. 249.
8. T. H. Morgan, *Evolution and Genetics* (Princeton: Princeton Univ. Press, 1915), pp. 206-7.
9. R. Pearl, "The biology of superiority," *American Mercury*, 1927, 47: 257-66.
10. W. Wolfensberger, "The extermination of handicapped people in World War II Germany," *Ment. Retard.*, 1981 (Feb.): 1-7.
11. E. A. Carlson, *Genes, Radiation, and Society* (Ithaca: Cornell Univ. Press, 1982), p. 179.
12. E. A. Hooton, "Human Heredity or Forbidden Fruit of the Tree of Knowledge," in *Medical Genetics and Eugenics*, vol. 2, ed. R. R. Gates et al. (Philadelphia: Women's Medical College of Pennsylvania, 1943), p. 53.
13. L. Ward, "Social Darwinism," *Am. J. Soc.*, 1907, 12: 693-716.
14. D. Freeman, *Margaret Mead and Samoa* (Suffolk: Pelican Books, 1985), pp. 24-26.
15. Ibid., p. 32.
16. Boas, *Changes in Bodily Form.*
17. M. Mead, *Coming of Age in Samoa* (New York: Morrow, 1928).
18. J. E. Coogan to Eugenics Record Office, Nov. 12, 1940, Davenport Papers, Laughlin box 20.
19. L. Penrose, *The Biology of Mental Defect* (London: Sidgwick and Jackson, 1949), p. 234.
20. Ibid.
21. S. L. Halpern, "Human heredity and mental deficiency," *Am. J. Ment. Def.*, 1947, 51: 153-63.
22. S. M. Donovan, "A Catholic, some eugenicists speak," *Eugenics*, 1930, 3 (no. 5): 181.
23. R. H. Johnson, "Legislation," *Eugenics*, 1927, 2 (no. 4): 64.
24. F. L. Broderick, *Right Reverend New Dealer: John A. Ryan* (New York: Macmillan, 1963), pp. 148-50.
25. J. Mayer, "Eugenics in Roman Catholic literature," *Eugenics*, 1930, 3 (no. 2): 43-51.
26. *Five Great Encyclicals* (New York: Paulist Press, 1939), pp. 96-97.
27. E. Schmiedeleer, *Sterilization in the United States* (Washington, D.C.: National Catholic Welfare Conference, 1943).
28. M. S. Olden, "Present status of sterilization legislation in the United States," *Eugenical News*, 1945, 30: 3-14.
29. Ibid., p. 13.
30. C. Pierson, "Are we sufficiently progressed scientifically for the legal sexual

sterilization of inmates of state institutions in certain cases?" *New Orleans Med. Surg. J.,* 1929, 82: 350-59.

31. W. Fernald, "After-care study of the patients discharged from Waverly for a period of twenty-five years," *Am. J. Ment. Def.,* 1919, 4: 62-81.
32. A. Myerson, "Some objections to sterilization," *Birth Control Rev.,* 1928, 12: 81-84.
33. A. Myerson and R. Elkind, "Researches in feeblemindedness," *Bull. Mass. Dept. Ment. Dis.,* 1930, 16: 108-229.
34. A. Myerson et al., *Eugenical Sterilization: A Reorientation of the Problem* (New York: Macmillan, 1936).
35. Ibid., p. 4.
36. Letter to C. Campbell, Feb. 12, 1936, Huntington Archives, box 30, folder 302.
37. Judge Frank Cooper to Dr. Harry Perkins, Feb. 12, 1936, Huntington Archives, box 30, folder 302.
38. A. Myerson, "Critique of proposed 'ideal' legislation," *Arch. Neur. Psy.,* 1935, 33: 453-66.
39. A. Myerson, "Research urged," Letter to the editor, *New York Times,* Mar. 15, 1936, Huntington Archives, box 30, folder 302.
40. Myerson et al., *Eugenical Sterilization.*
41. J. H. Landman, "Race betterment by human sterilization," *Sci. Am.,* 1934, 150: 292-95.
42. E. S. Gosney, "Eugenical sterilization," *Sci. Am.,* 1934, 150: 18-22.
43. C. Thomalla, "The sterilization law in Germany," *Sci. Am.,* 1934, 150: 118-22.
44. I. Cox, "The folly of human sterilization," *Sci. Am.,* 1934, 150: 188-90.
45. J. C. Merriam to H.H.L., Dec. 31, 1938, Davenport Archives, Laughlin folder 37.
46. "Sterilization of criminals," *Fortune,* 1937 (June): 106.
47. "Finishing schools," *Time,* Nov. 8, 1937, p. 15.
48. J. H. Kempton, "Sterilization for ten million Americans," *J. Heredity,* 1935, 26: 415-18.
49. A. E. Wiggam, *The New Decalogue of Science* (Indianapolis: Bobbs-Merrill, 1923).
50. G. S. Hall to G. Drank, Undated, Davenport Archives, Laughlin folder 20.
51. A. E. Wiggam, *The Fruit of the Family Tree* (Indianapolis: Bobbs-Merrill, 1924), p. 334.
52. A. E. Wiggam, *The Next Age of Man* (Indianapolis: Bobbs-Merrill, 1927), p. 355.
53. L. C. Dunn and T. Dobzhansky, *Heredity, Race, and Society* (New York: New American Library, 1952), pp. 90-94.
54. C. Gamble, "Preventive sterilization in 1948," *JAMA,* 1949, 141: 773.

Chapter 9: The Quiet Years

1. *Skinner v. Oklahoma,* 316 U.S. 535 (1942).
2. M. A. Taromianz to the New Jersey Sterilization League (NJSL), May 7, 1944, AVS Archives, folder 58.
3. M. L. Perry to NJSL, May 4, 1945, AVS Archives, folder 59.

4. "Pope again denounces sterilization of humans," *New York Herald Tribune,* Sept. 8, 1953, AVS Archives, folder 13.
5. The material on the New Jersey Sterilization League and Marion S. Norton is based on my review of the AVS Archives.
6. See the collection of letters from New Jersey legislators to M. S. Norton, Dec. 1935, AVS Archives, folder 3.
7. Minutes of NJSL meetings during 1937, AVS Archives, folder 1.
8. Minutes of NJSL meetings during 1938, AVS Archives, folder 1.
9. "Model sterilization law," Manuscript, 1941 or 1942, AVS Archives, folder 4.
10. R. C. Hardy to NJSL, Apr. 11, 1942, AVS Archives, folder 4.
11. Resignation of Marion Norton, Jan. 1943, AVS Archives, folder 2.
12. Minutes of organizational meeting of Birthright, Inc., Apr. 12, 1943, AVS Archives, folder 7.
13. Report of the Field Committee of Birthright, Dec. 1946, AVS Archives, folder 10.
14. Minutes of Executive Committee of Birthright, Apr. 11, 1947, AVS Archives, folder 7.
15. "Sterilization officially reported up to January 1, 1950, from states having a sterilization law," AVS Archives, Unnumbered folder.
16. F. O. Butler and C. J. Gamble, "Sterilization in a California School for the mentally deficient," *Am. J. Ment. Def.,* 1947, 51 (no. 4): 745-47.
17. C. Gamble, "Preventive sterilization in 1948," *JAMA,* 1949, 141 (no. 11): 773.
18. "State sterilization," *Newsweek,* Nov. 28, 1949; "For fewer unfit," *Newsweek,* Oct. 30, 1950.
19. L. L. Stanley to NJSL, Feb. 3, 1940, AVS Archives, folder 55.
20. F. O. Butler to NJSL, May 3, 1947. AVS Archives, folder 61.
21. L. L. Stanley to AVS, Apr. 21, 1950, AVS Archives, folder 69.
22. See replies to annual sterilization surveys for 1949 and 1950 conducted by Birthright, AVS Archives, folders 76-81.The letters are dated June 13, 1950 (Indiana); June 15, 1950 (Georgia); and Feb. 7, 1951 (Virginia).
23. See replies to annual sterilization surveys for 1948, 1949, and 1955, AVS Archives, folders 76-81. Letters are dated Jan. 11, 1949 (S. Dakota); Apr. 20, 1950 (Missouri); and Jan. 3, 1956 (Indiana).
24. Report of Dr. F. O. Butler, Dec. 1, 1950, AVS Archives, folder 11.
25. Human Betterment League of Iowa, 1949, Press Release: "72,771 years saved by sterilization in California," AVS Archives, folder 16.
26. "Dr. Butler's reports on field trips and other activities from September 27 through December 15, 1949," AVS Archives, folder 20.
27. W. S. Hall to AVS, Jan. 4, 1956, AVS Archives, folder 81.
28. Woodside, *Sterilization in North Carolina.*
29. "Sterilizations performed in the year 1948 by Eugenics Board of North Carolina," Jan. 7, 1949, AVS Archives, folder 64.
30. Eugenics Board of North Carolina to Human Betterment Association of America, Jan. 15, 1963, AVS Archives, Unnumbered folder.
31. Human Betterment League of North Carolina, Form letter, AVS Archives, folder 18.
32. E. Speas to AVS, Mar. 19, 1956, AVS Archives, folder 84.
33. M. Thompson, *Prologue: A Minnesota Story of Mental Retardation* (Minneapolis: Gilbert, 1963).

34. Ibid., p. 57.
35. Ibid., p. 59.
36. State Board of Control of Minnesota, *Thirteenth Biennial Report.*
37. Interview with Arthur Madow, Faribault, Minnesota, Nov. 11, 1982.
38. State Board of Control of Minnesota, *Twenty-Fourth Biennial Report* (Stillwater, Minnesota: State Prison Printing Dept., 1948).
39. Ibid., p. 64.
40. Thompson, *Prologue,* p. 142.
41. Ibid., pp. 182-83.
42. Interview with Madow.
43. Interview with Dean Nelson, Faribault, Minnesota, Nov. 11, 1982.
44. This material is based on records in the office of Dr. Madow. I do not further identify it out of respect for patient privacy.
45. Memorandum from Dr. David Vail. This was provided to me by Arthur Madow, Nov. 11, 1982.
46. Interview with Madow.
47. *Howard v. Des Moines Register & Tribune Co.,* 283 N.W. 2nd 289 (1979).
48. Letter from Clifford Forster (Acting Director, ACLU), May 7, 1947, AVS Archives, folder 14.
49. "Catholic hospital bids 7 doctors quit birth control unit or leave," *New York Herald Tribune,* Feb. 1, 1952, AVS Archives, folder 94.
50. L. K. Champlin and M. F. Winslow, "Elective sterilization," *U. Penn. Law Rev.,* 1965, 113 (no. 3): 415-44.
51. B. H. Singer to AVS, Apr. 17, 1957, AVS Archives, folder 21.
52. Memorandum, "For physicians concerned with voluntary sterilization," Apr. 1960, AVS Archives, folder 23.
53. *Operation for Purposes of Human Sterilization,* Bulletin of the Joint Commission on Accreditation of Hospitals, Dec. 1961, AVS Archives, folder 24.
54. "Aid for sterilization program is discussed," *Lexington Herald,* May 30, 1961, AVS Archives, folder 99.
55. "50 indigent mothers sterilized in Fauquier County," *Washington Post,* Sept. 4, 1962, AVS Archives, folder 100.
56. "O'Boyle assails sterilization," *Washington Star,* Sept. 10, 1962, AVS Archives, folder 100.
57. "Virginians calm on sterilization," *New York Times,* Sept. 12, 1962, AVS Archives, folder 100.
58. "Sterilization: new argument," *U.S. News & World Report,* Sept. 24, 1962, AVS Archives, folder 101.
59. "$25,000 fund starts sterilization plan," *Boston Globe,* July 9, 1964, AVS Archives, folder 102.
60. "Sterilization bill favored by judge," *Raleigh News & Observer,* Apr. 20, 1963, AVS Archives, folder 102.
61. J. Paul, "The return of punitive sterilization laws," *Law & Soc. Policy,* 1970, 1: 1-64.
62. Memorandum, "Operation Lawsuit—status," Mar. 20, 1970, AVS Archives, folder 2.
63. "Hospitals refusing to perform sterilization operations hit in suits," *Harrisburg News,* Dec. 28, 1971, AVS Archives, folder 1.
64. *Roe v. Wade,* 410 U.S. 113, 1973.

Chapter 10: Involuntary Sterilization Today

1. F. T. Landman and D. M. McIntyre, Jr., eds., *The Mentally Disabled and the Law* (Chicago: University of Chicago Press, 1961), pp. 183-97.
2. J. A. Varner, "Rights of mentally ill—involuntary sterilization—analysis of recent statutes," *W. Virg. Law Rev.,* 1975, 78: 131-42.
3. *Holmes v. Powers,* 439 S.W. 2d 579 (1968).
4. *Frazier v. Levi,* 440 S.W. 2d 393 (1969).
5. *In re Cavitt,* 157 N.W. 2d 171 (1968).
6. *North Carolina Association for Retarded Children v. North Carolina,* 420 F. Supp. 451 (1976).
7. *Wyatt v. Aderholt,* 368 F. Supp. 1382 (1973).
8. Telephone interview with J. J. Levin, Jr., Washington, D.C., Jan. 22, 1983.
9. *Relf v. Weinberger,* 372 F. Supp. 1196 (1974).
10. *Relf v. Matthews,* 403 F. Supp. 1235 (1975).
11. *Relf v. Weinberger,* 565 F. 2d 722 (1977).
12. *Federal Register,* Nov. 8, 1978, 43 (no. 217): 52146-75.
13. *Cook v. State,* 495 P. 2d 768 (1972).
14. *In re Moore,* 289 N.C. 95, 221 S.E. 2d 307 (1976).
15. E.P.C. Vining and J. M. Freeman, "Sterilization and the retarded female: is advocacy depriving individuals of their rights?" *Pediatrics,* 1978, 62 (no. 5): 850-52.
16. *Interest of M.K.R.,* 515 S.W. 2d 467 (1974); *A.L. v. G.R.H.,* 325 N.E.2d 501 (1975); *Guardianship of Tulley,* 146 Cal. Rptr. 64 (1974); *In the Matter of S.C.E.,* 378 A. 2d 144 (1977); *Hudson v. Hudson,* 373 So. 2d 310 (1979); *In re Flanary,* 6 Fam. L. Rep. 2345 (1980).
17. *Sparkman v. McFarlin,* 552 F. 2d 172 (1977).
18. *In the Matter of S.C.E.,* 378 A. 2d 144 (1977).
19. *Stump v. Sparkman,* 435 U.S. 349 (1978).
20. *In re Marcia R.,* 383 A. 2d 630 (1978).
21. *Ruby v. Massey,* 452 F. Supp. 361 (1978).
22. *In the Matter of Grady,* 426 N.E. 2d 467 (1981).
23. *Poe v. Lynchburg,* 518 F. Supp. 789 (1981).
24. Eliot Mincberg, Esq., to the author, Sept. 16, 1982.
25. Office of Virginia governor John Dalton, Press Release, Feb. 29, 1980.
26. P. C. McQueen et al., "Causal origins of major mental handicap in the Canadian maritime provinces," *Devel. Med. Child Neurol.,* 1986, 28: 697-707.
27. H. W. Moser and P. A. Wolf, *The Nosology of Mental Retardation,* Birth Defects Original Article Series, vol. 8, no. 1 (Feb. 1971), pp. 117-34.
28. J.B.S. Haldane, *Heredity and Politics* (New York: Norton, 1938), pp. 92-93.
29. E. W. Reed and S. C. Reed, *Mental Retardation: A Family Study* (Philadelphia: Saunders, 1965).
30. L. M. Spano and J. M. Opitz, "Bibliography on X-linked mental retardation, the fragile X, and related subjects IV," *Am. J. Med. Gen.,* 1988, 30: 51-60.
31. J. Paul, "The return of punitive sterilization proposals," *Law & Society Rev.,* 1968, 4: 77-110.
32. "Official urges sterilization of Texas welfare recipients," *New York Times,* Feb. 28, 1980.
33. *American Medical News,* Sept. 8, 1978, p. 22.

34. *Texas Observer,* Mar. 20, 1981.
35. *Boston Globe,* Mar. 31, 1982.
36. S. A. Mednick and K. O. Christiansen, eds., *Biosocial Bases of Criminal Behavior* (New York: Gardner Press, 1977).
37. P. A. Jacobs et al., "Chromosome studies in men in a maximum security hospital," *Ann. Hum. Gen.,* 1968, 31: 339-42.
38. *Oil, Chemical and Atomic Workers v. American Cyanamid Co.,* 741 F. 2d 444 (1984).
39. Office of Technology Assessment, *The Role of Genetic Testing in the Prevention of Occupational Disease* (Washington, D.C.: GPO, 1983).
40. *Doerr v. Goodrich,* 484 F. Supp. 320 (1979).
41. P. R. Reilly, "Screening Workers: Privacy, Procreation, and Prevention," in *Reproduction: The New Frontier in Occupational and Environmental Health Research,* ed. J. E. Lockey et al. (New York: Liss, 1984), pp. 1-11.
42. "Women get access to jobs with rule," *New York Times,* May 19, 1990.
43. A. Chakravarti, "Compulsory Sterilization: A Valid Population Policy? or, Carrie Buck goes to India," Manuscript. The author interviewed Mr. Chakravarti about his research on Feb. 5, 1981, in Houston, Texas.
44. "China's one-child population future," *Intercom,* 1981, 9 (no. 8): 1, 12-14.
45. Ibid.
46. "Officials debate asylum for Chinese fleeing abortion policy," *New York Times,* Apr. 3, 1989.
47. "Chinese region uses new law to sterilize mentally retarded," *New York Times,* Nov. 21, 1989, p. 1.

Index